Pops, Don't Forget!

Pops, Don't Forget!

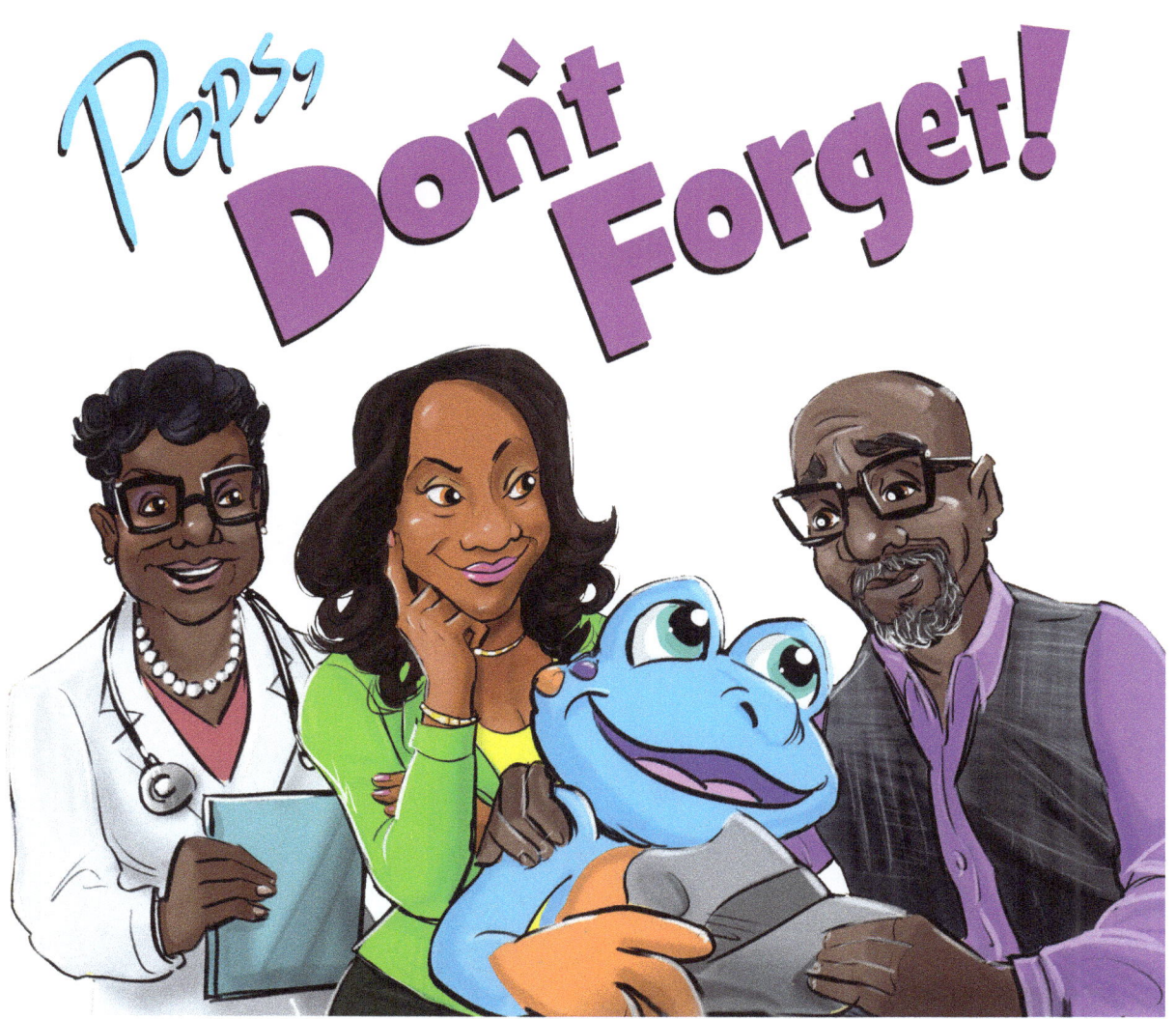

written by
Xylina Cassandra

Illustrated by
Rickey Boyd

Copyright 2025 by Xylina Cassandra. All rights reserved.

No portion of this book may be reproduced in any form without written permission from the publisher or author, except as permitted by U.S. copyright law.

ISBN: 979-8-9920951-4-2
ISBN: 979-8-9920951-3-5
ISBN: 979-8-9920951-5-9

Boss Frog LLC
www.bossfrog.com
Trademarked

www.BossFrog.org

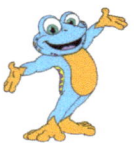

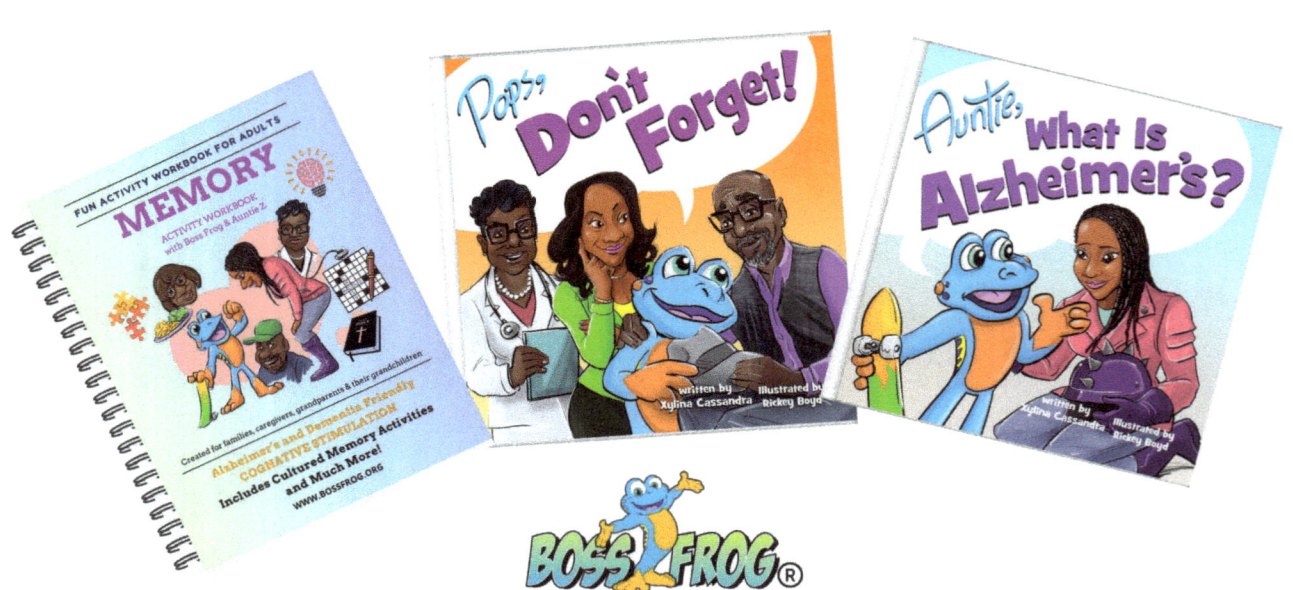

www.BossFrog.org

"Pops, Don't Forget!" – A Message on Dementia Awareness for Youth

Alzheimer's disease and other forms of dementia are silently but powerfully affecting the African American community. It's time we bring awareness to people of all ages, especially our youth. Young people often play important roles in caregiving and supporting older family members. By educating them about dementia, we empower them to recognize early signs and respond with compassion. This knowledge not only reduces shame and stigma—it opens the door to real conversations within our families.

This is why I'm so excited for the world to read *"Pops, Don't Forget!"* This book shows how children are often the first to notice memory changes in their grandparents. Their observations matter. We must listen—and we must educate! Together, we can help our youth lead the way to a healthier, more informed future for our families and communities.

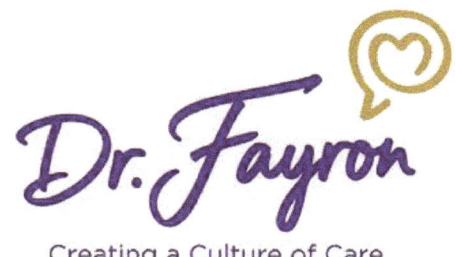

Fayron Epps, PhD, RN

Professor | Karen & Ronald Herrmann Distinguished Chair in Caregiving Research
UT Health San Antonio
School of Nursing

Pops, Don't Forget!

Xylina Cassandra

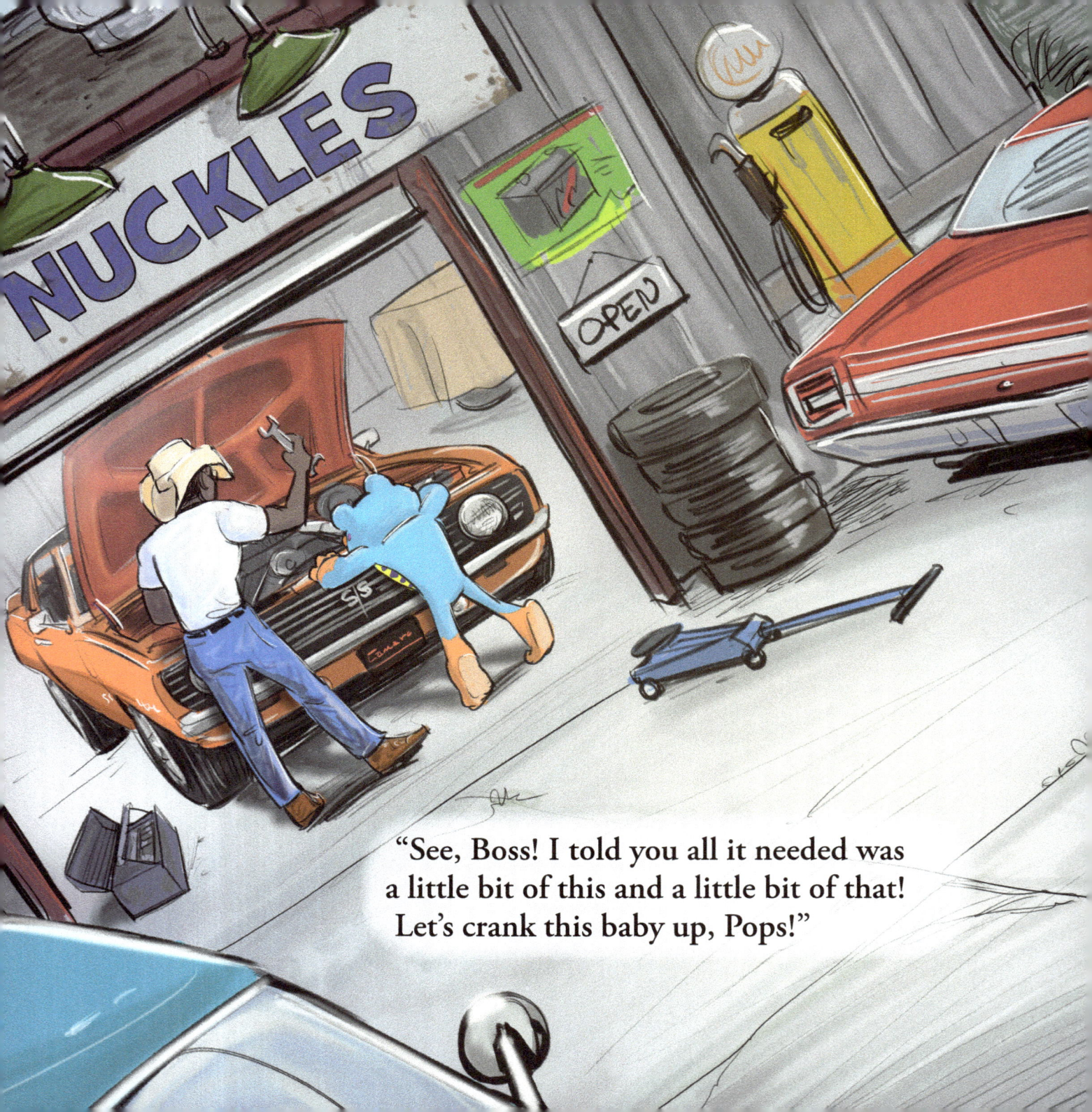

"See, Boss! I told you all it needed was a little bit of this and a little bit of that! Let's crank this baby up, Pops!"

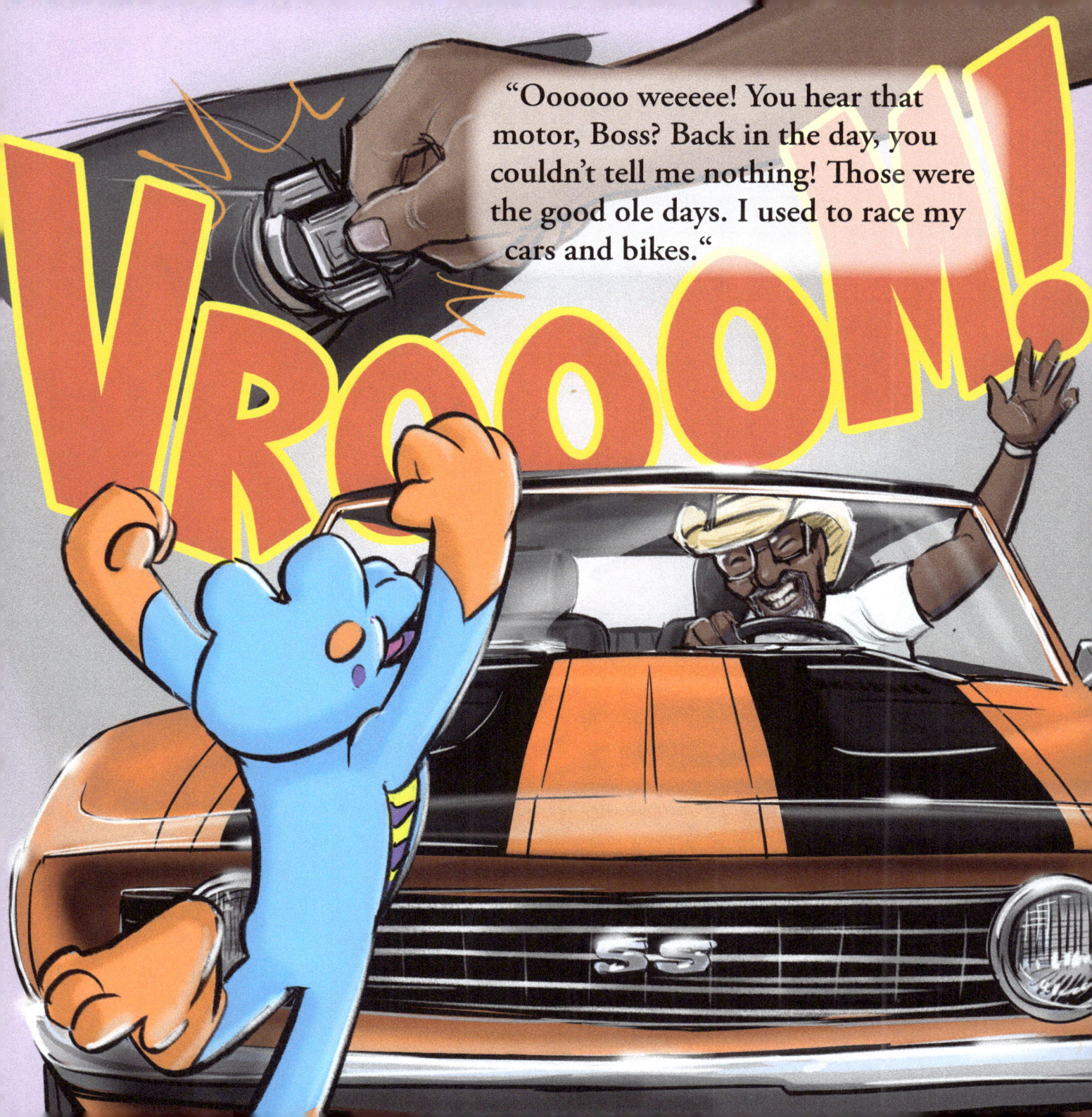

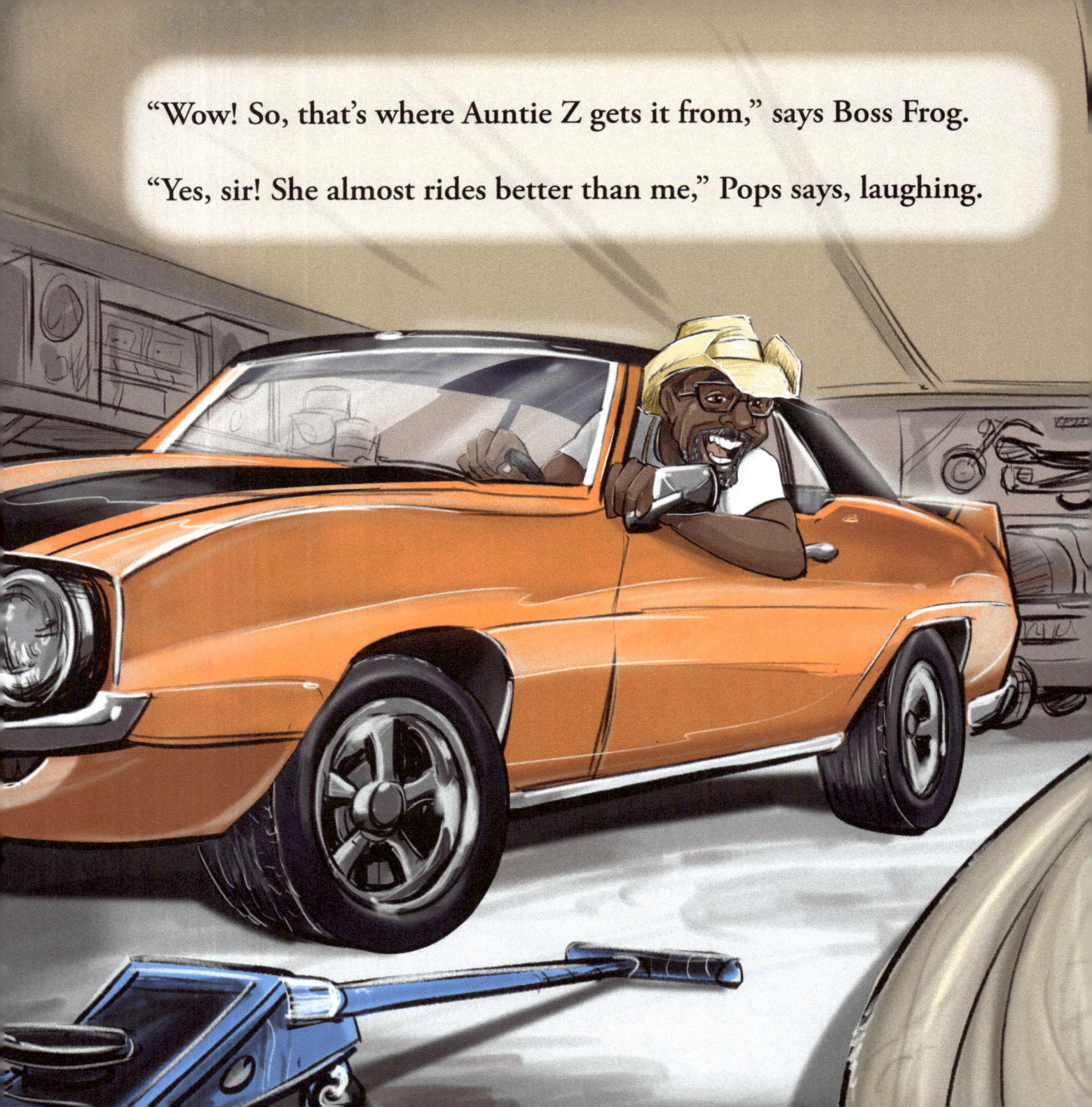

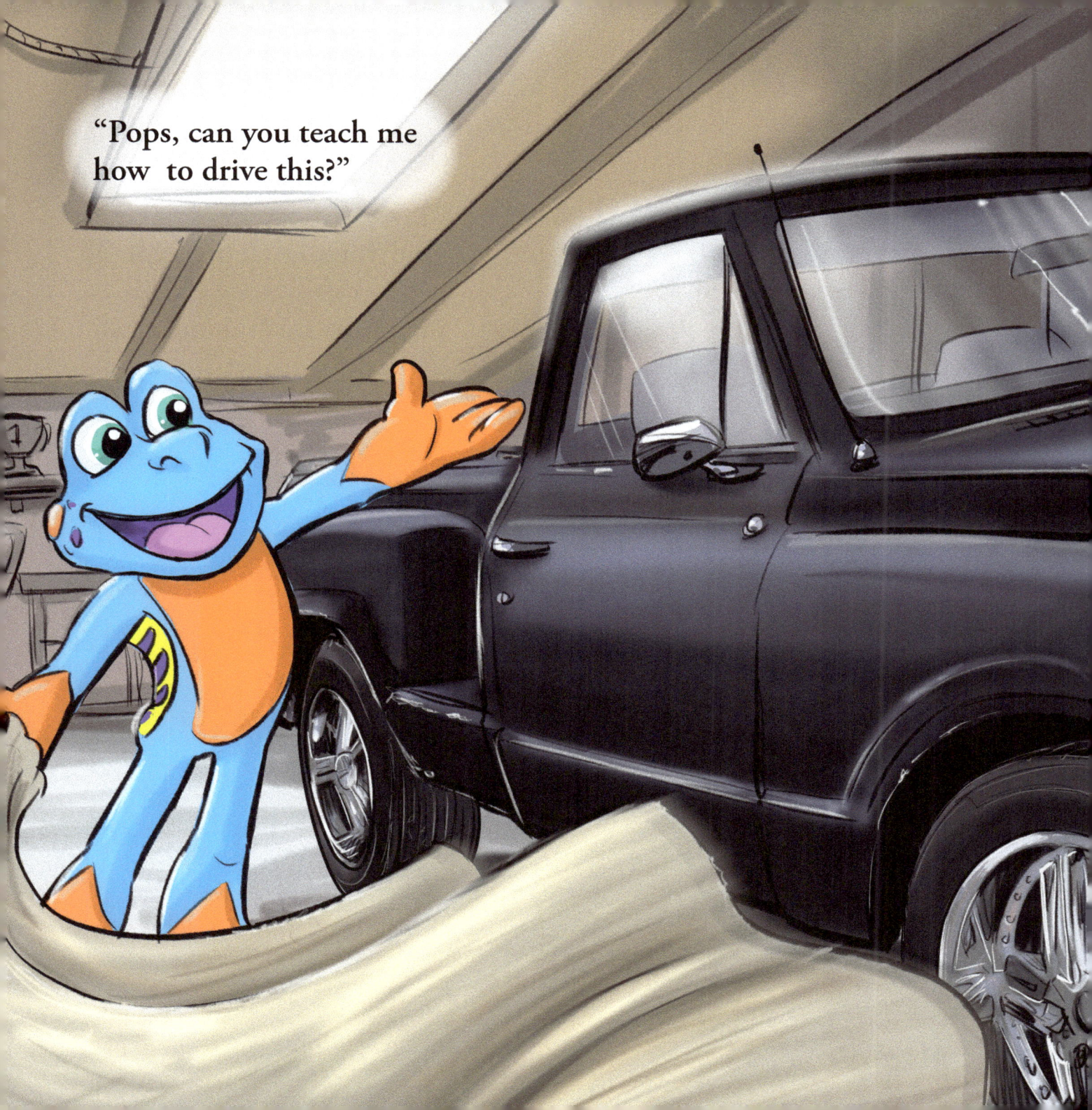

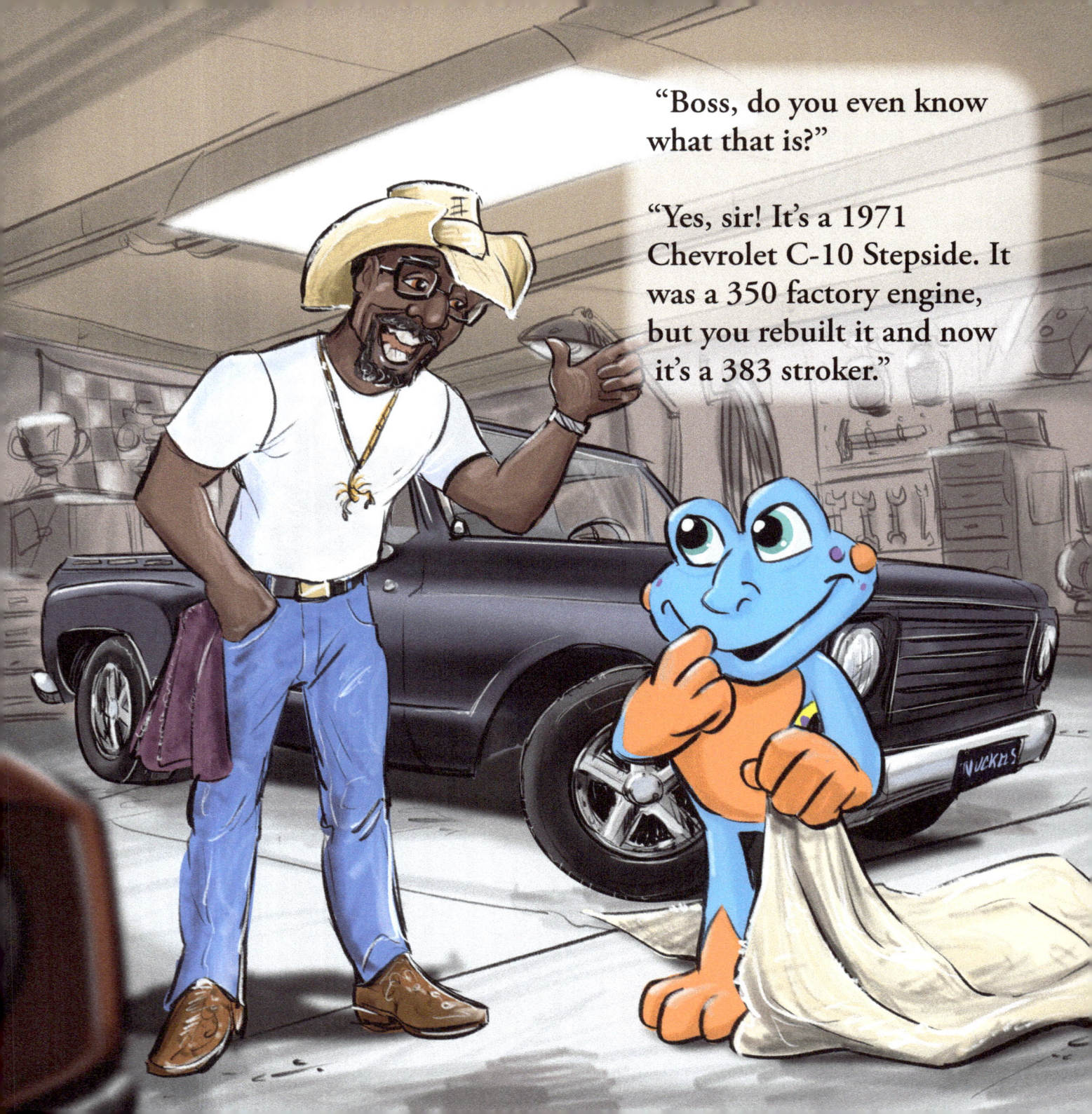

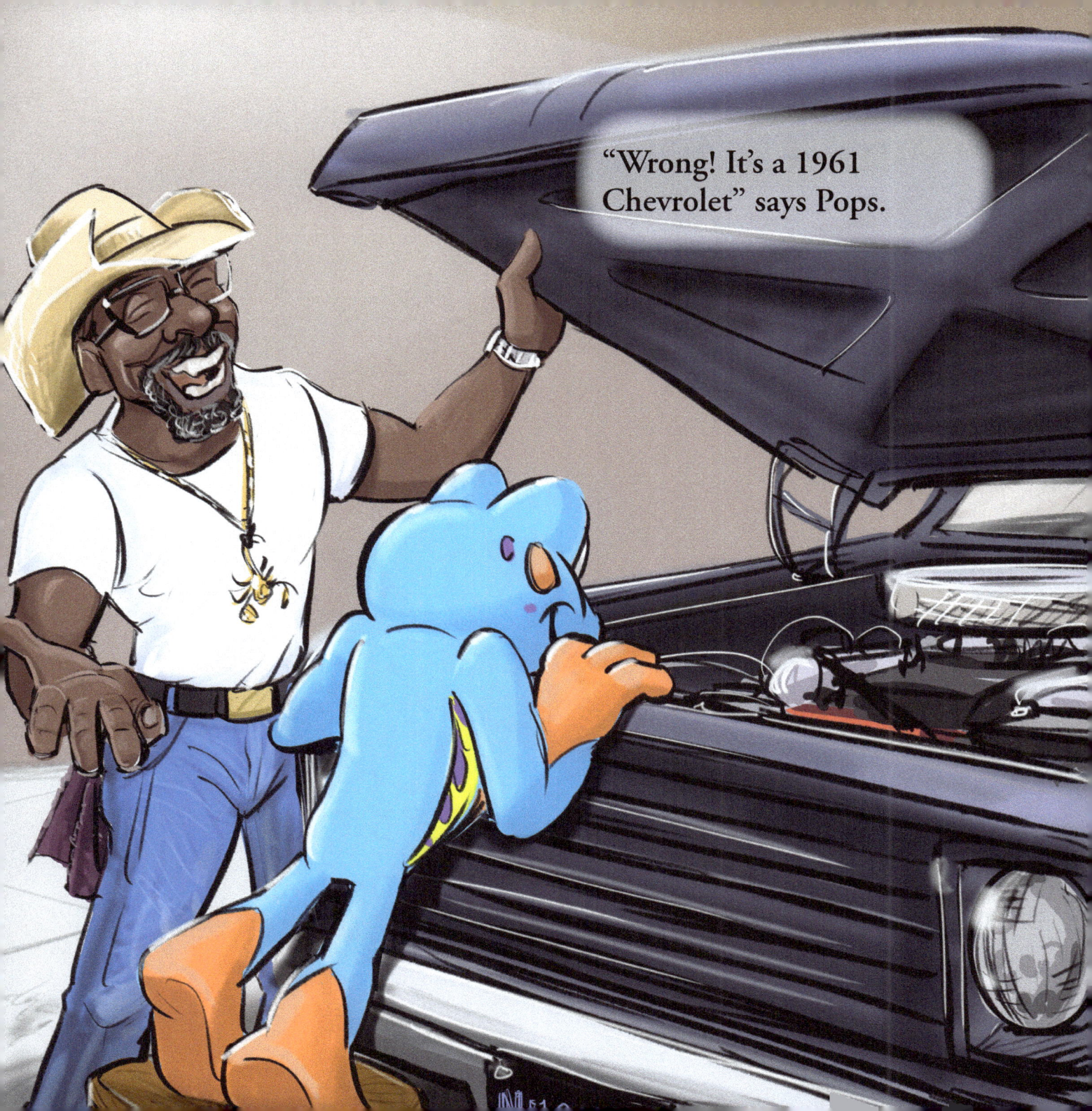

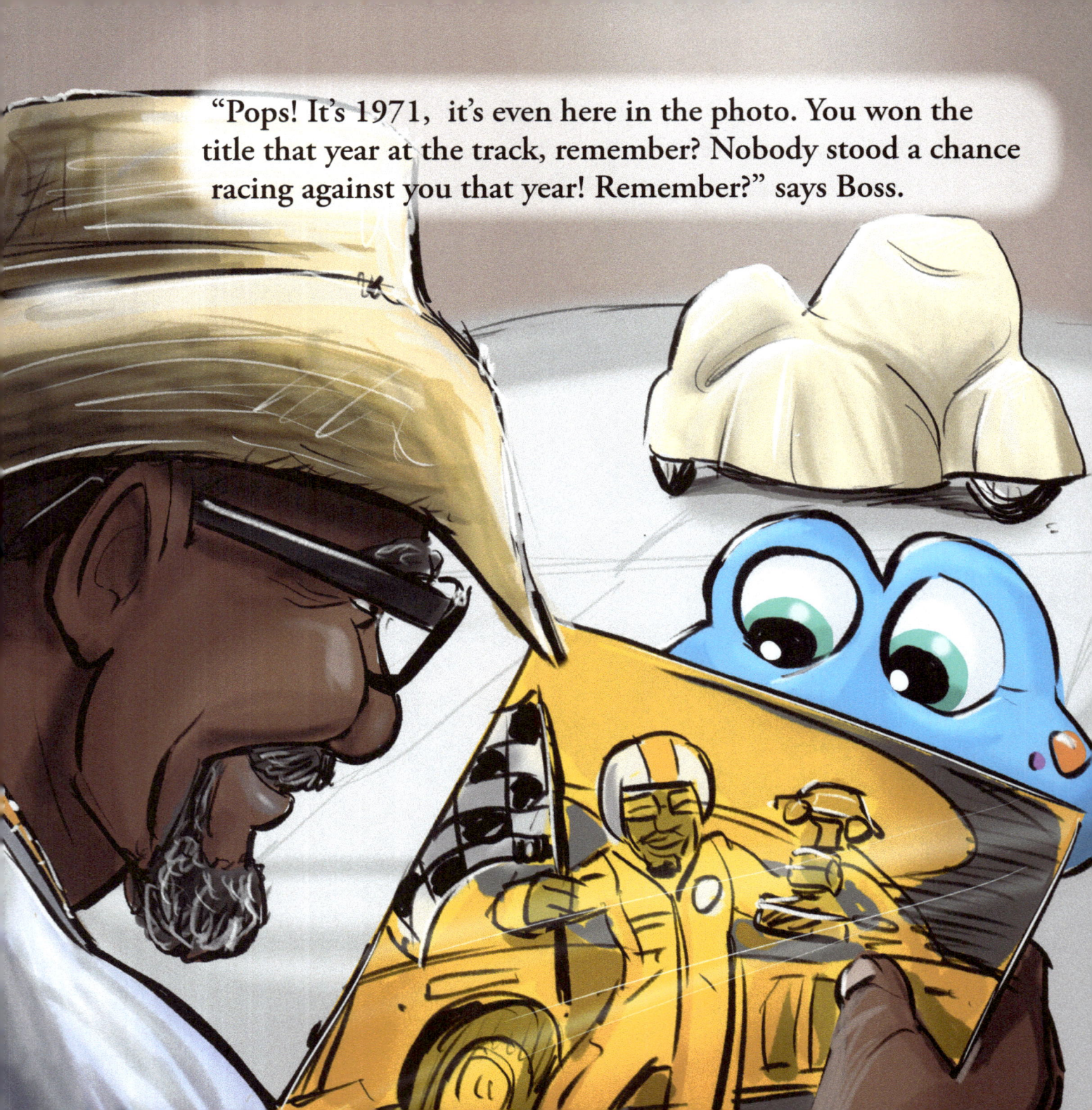

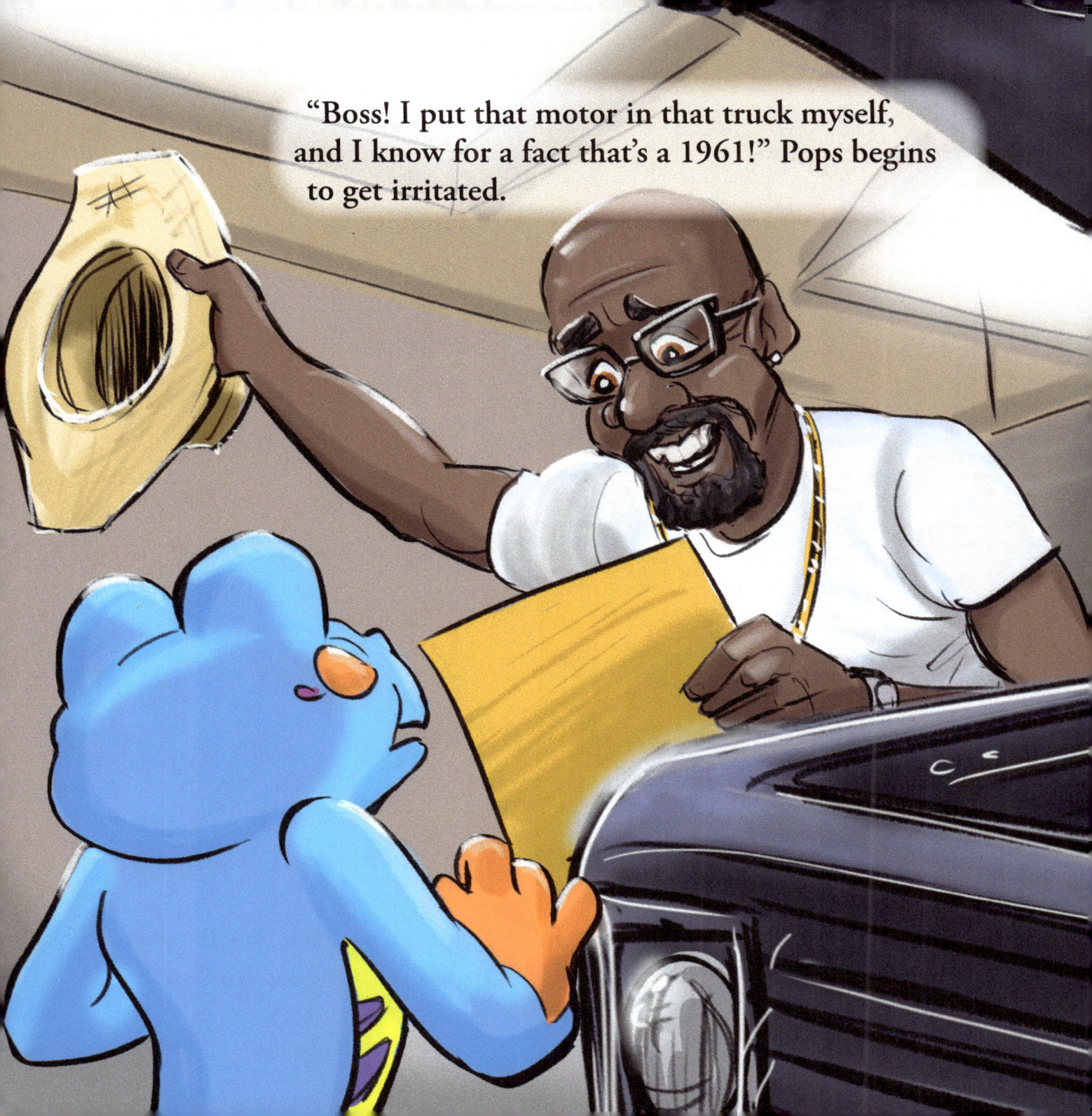

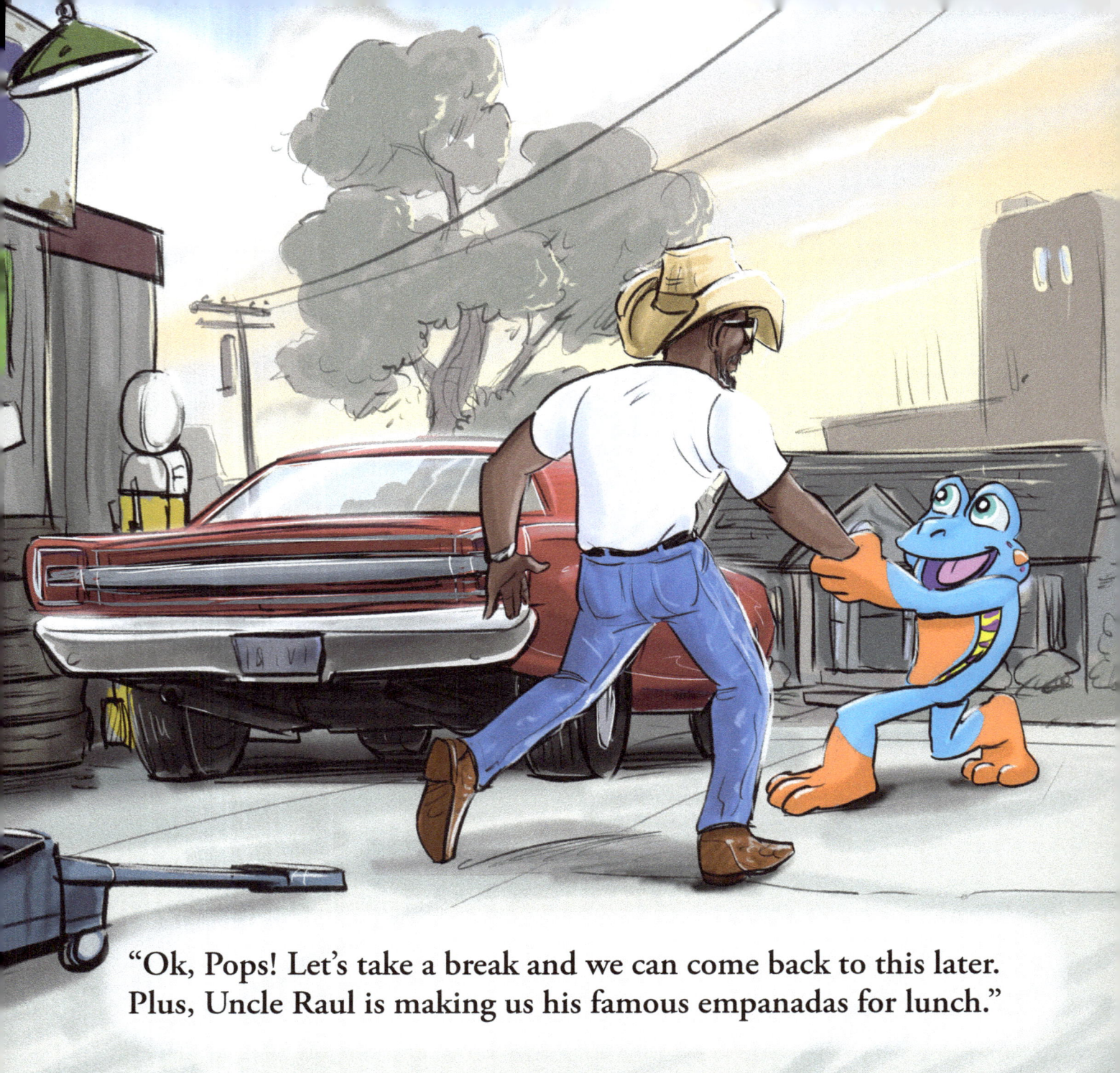

"Ok, Pops! Let's take a break and we can come back to this later. Plus, Uncle Raul is making us his famous empanadas for lunch."

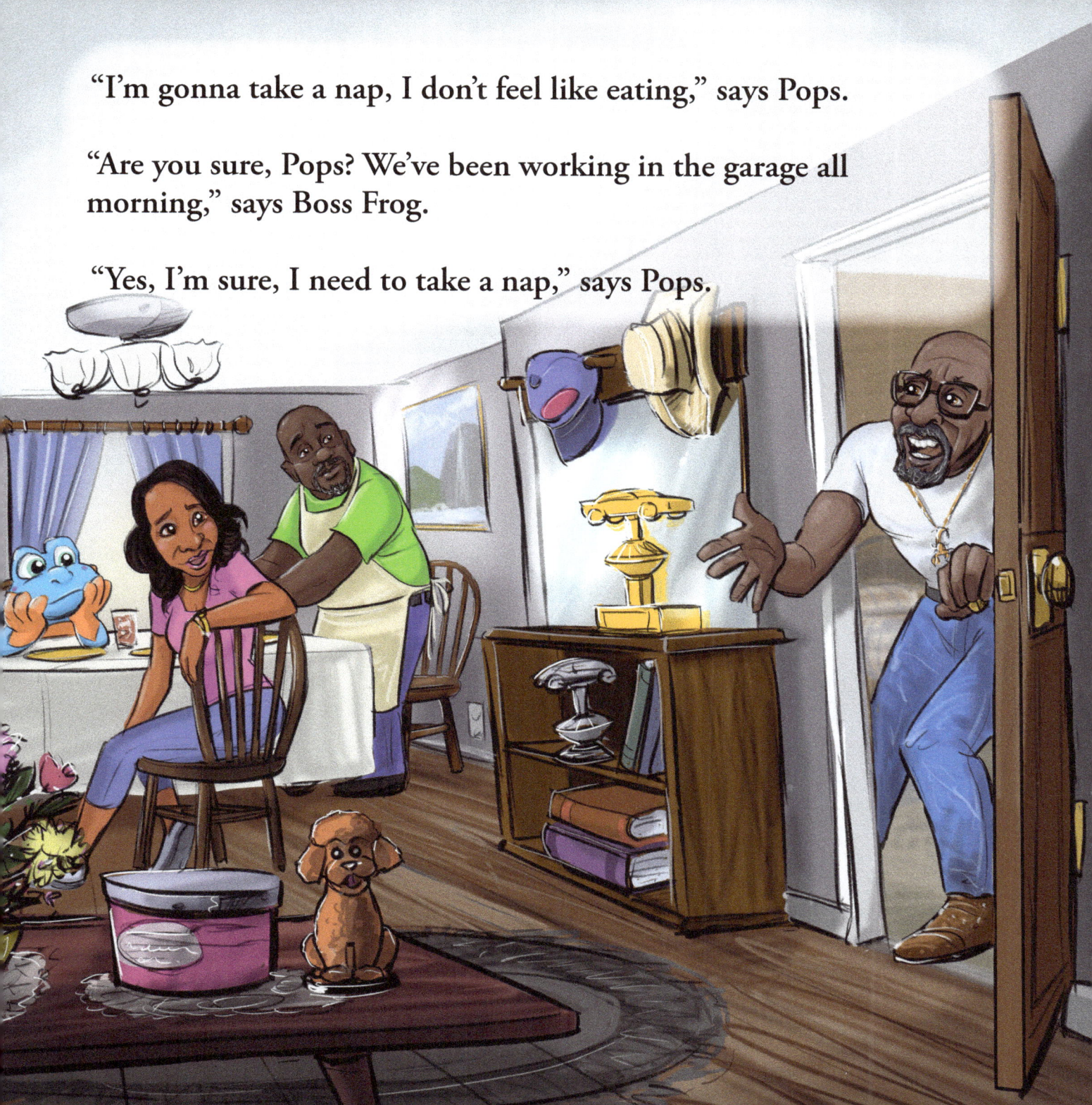

"I'm gonna take a nap, I don't feel like eating," says Pops.

"Are you sure, Pops? We've been working in the garage all morning," says Boss Frog.

"Yes, I'm sure, I need to take a nap," says Pops.

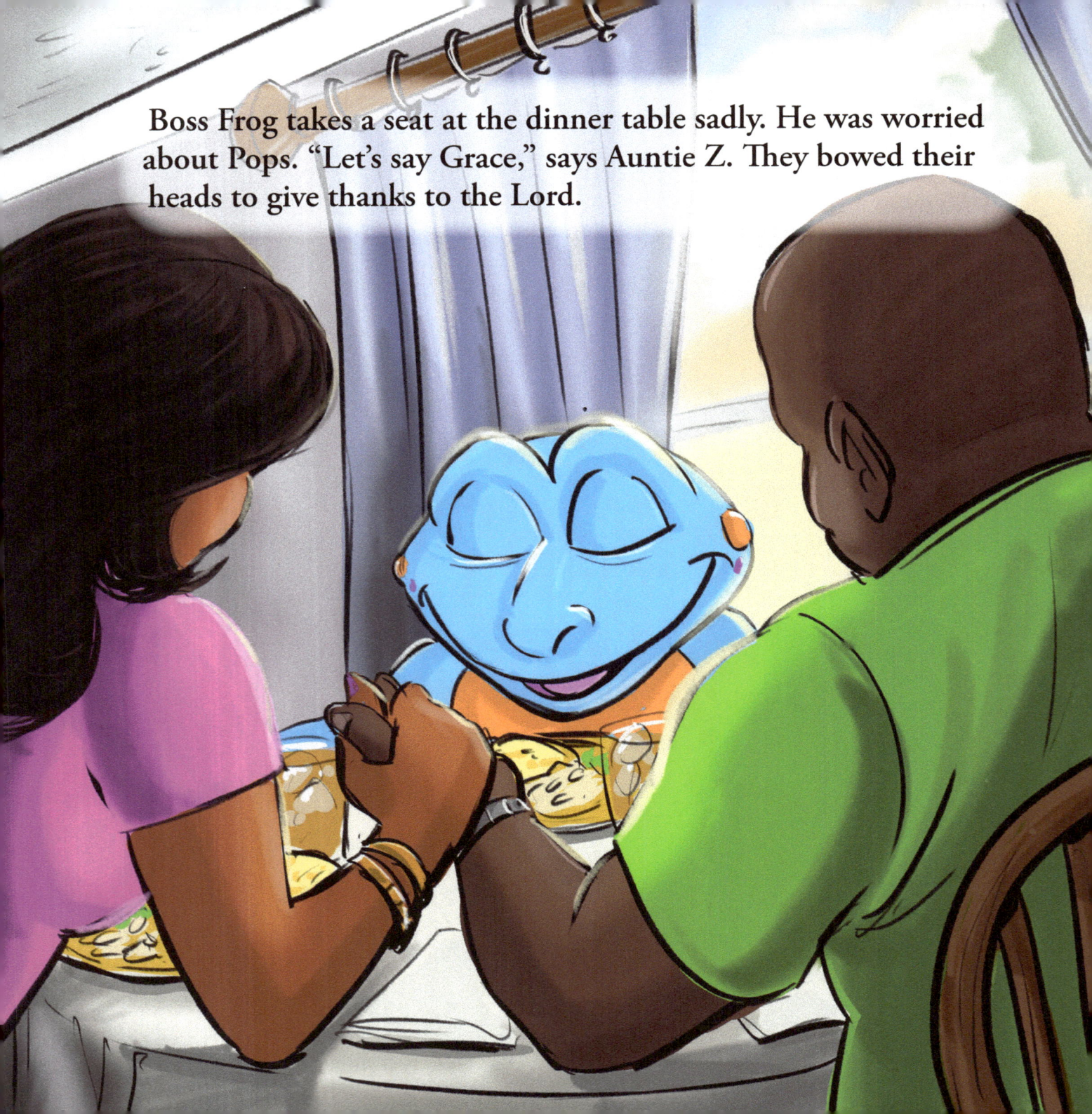

Boss Frog takes a seat at the dinner table sadly. He was worried about Pops. "Let's say Grace," says Auntie Z. They bowed their heads to give thanks to the Lord.

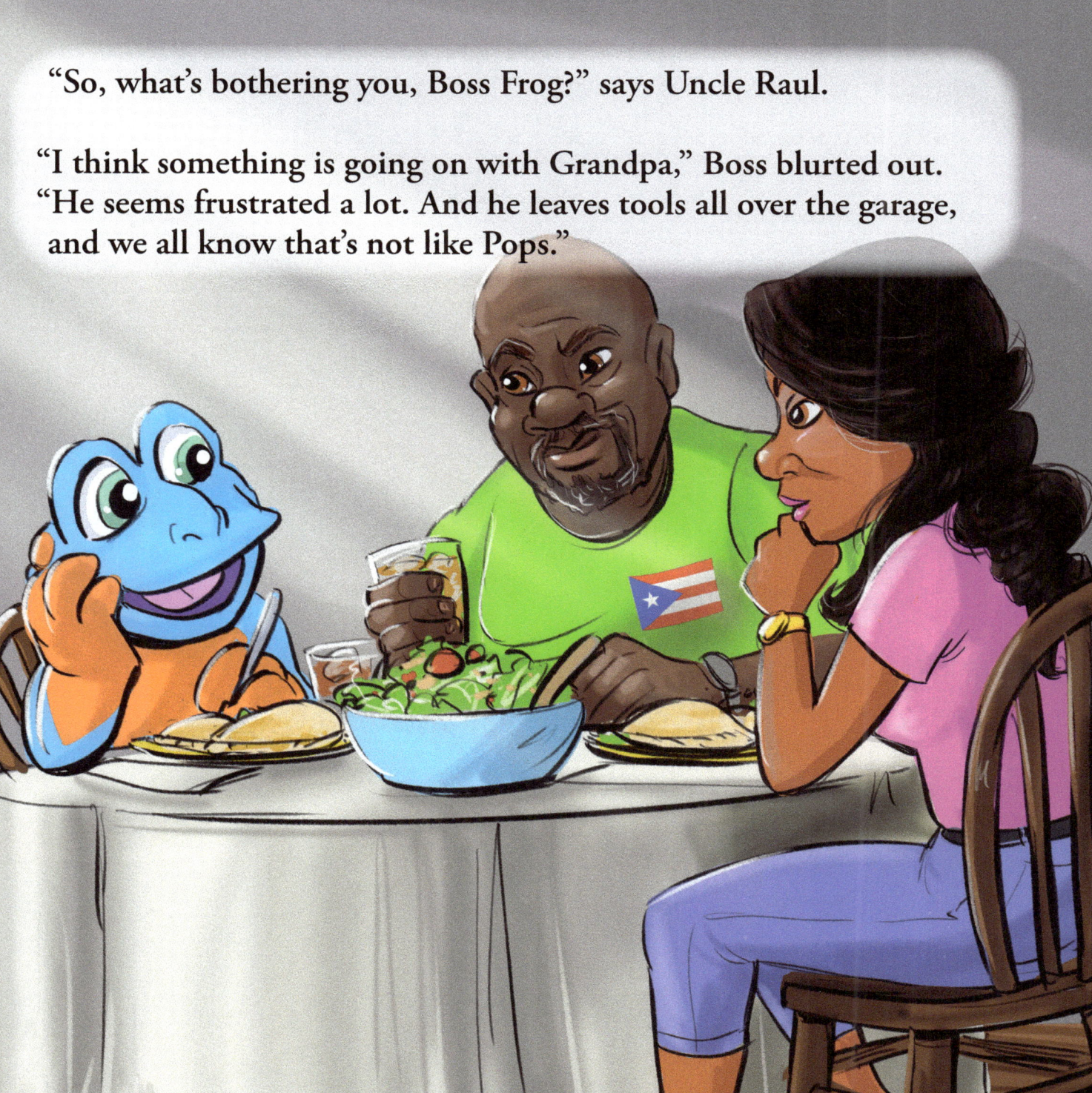

"So, what's bothering you, Boss Frog?" says Uncle Raul.

"I think something is going on with Grandpa," Boss blurted out. "He seems frustrated a lot. And he leaves tools all over the garage, and we all know that's not like Pops."

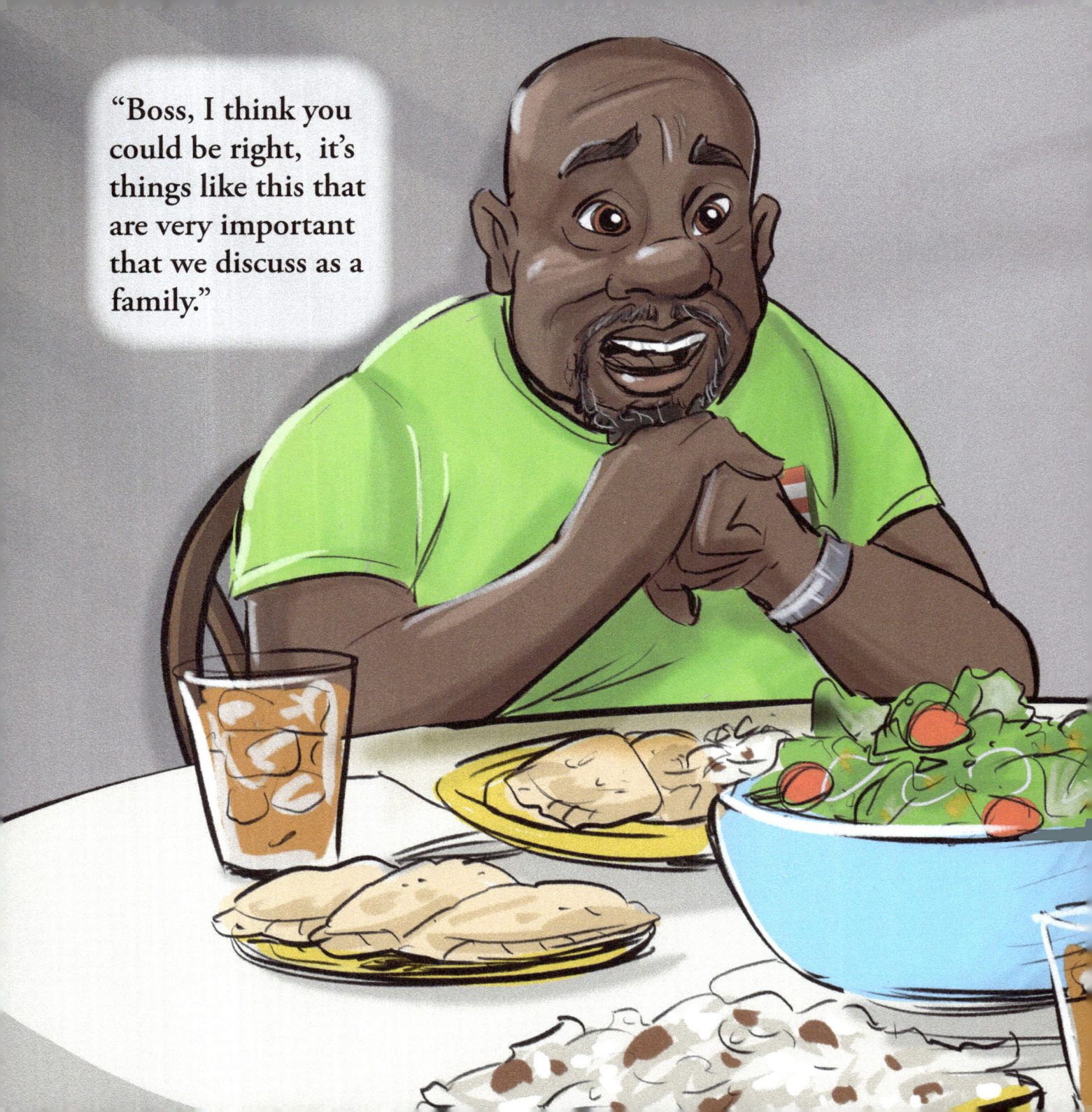

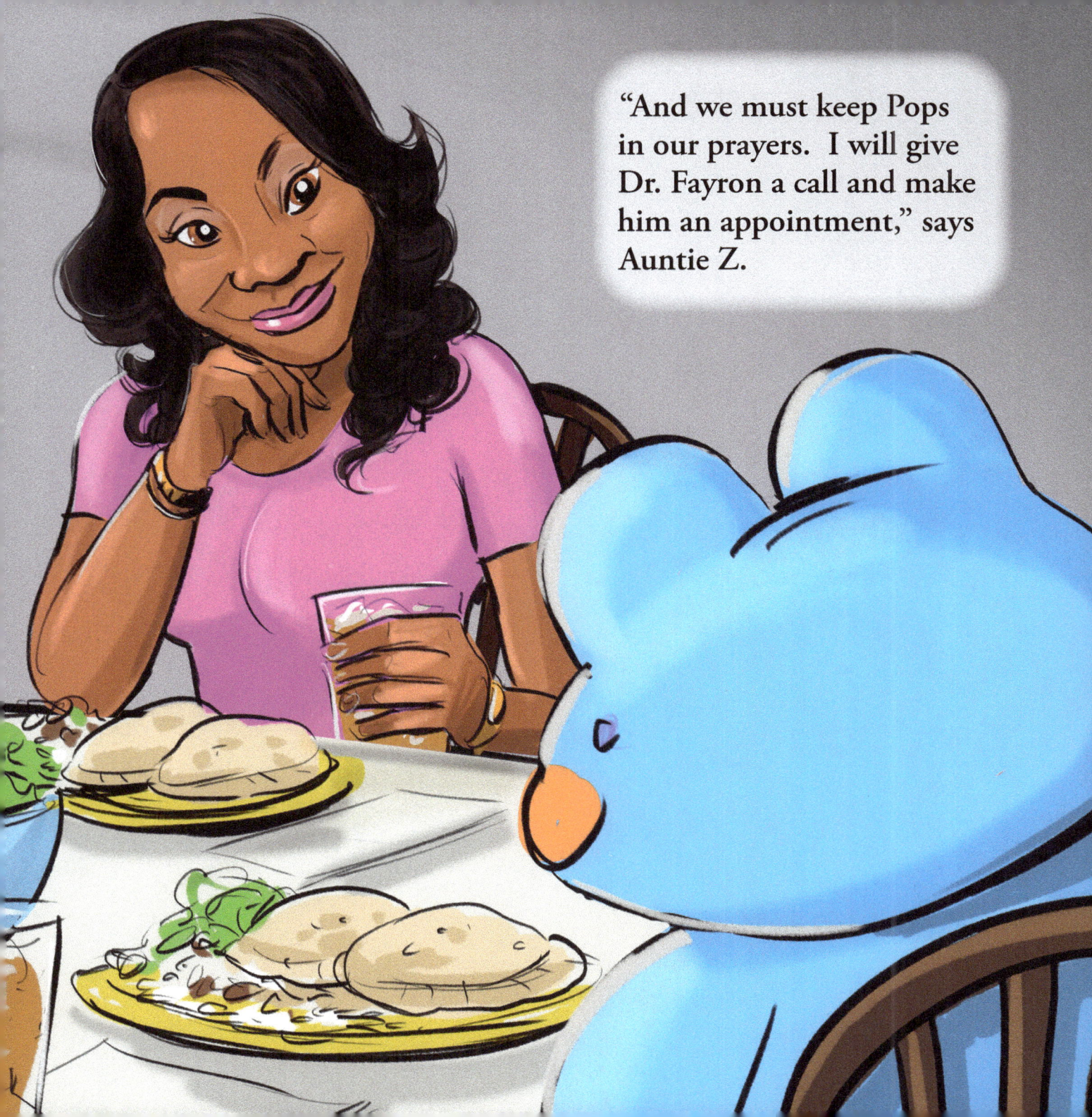

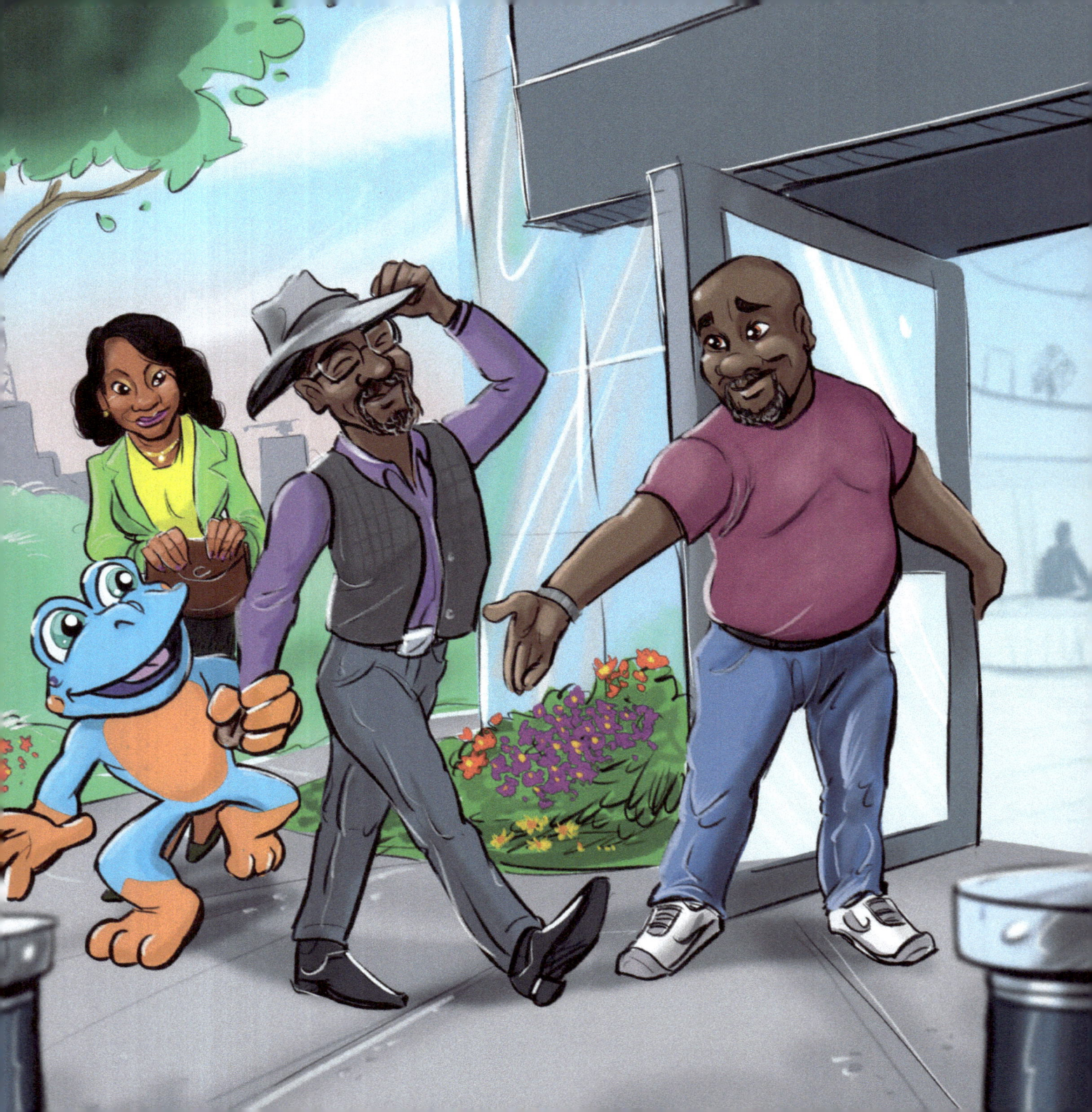

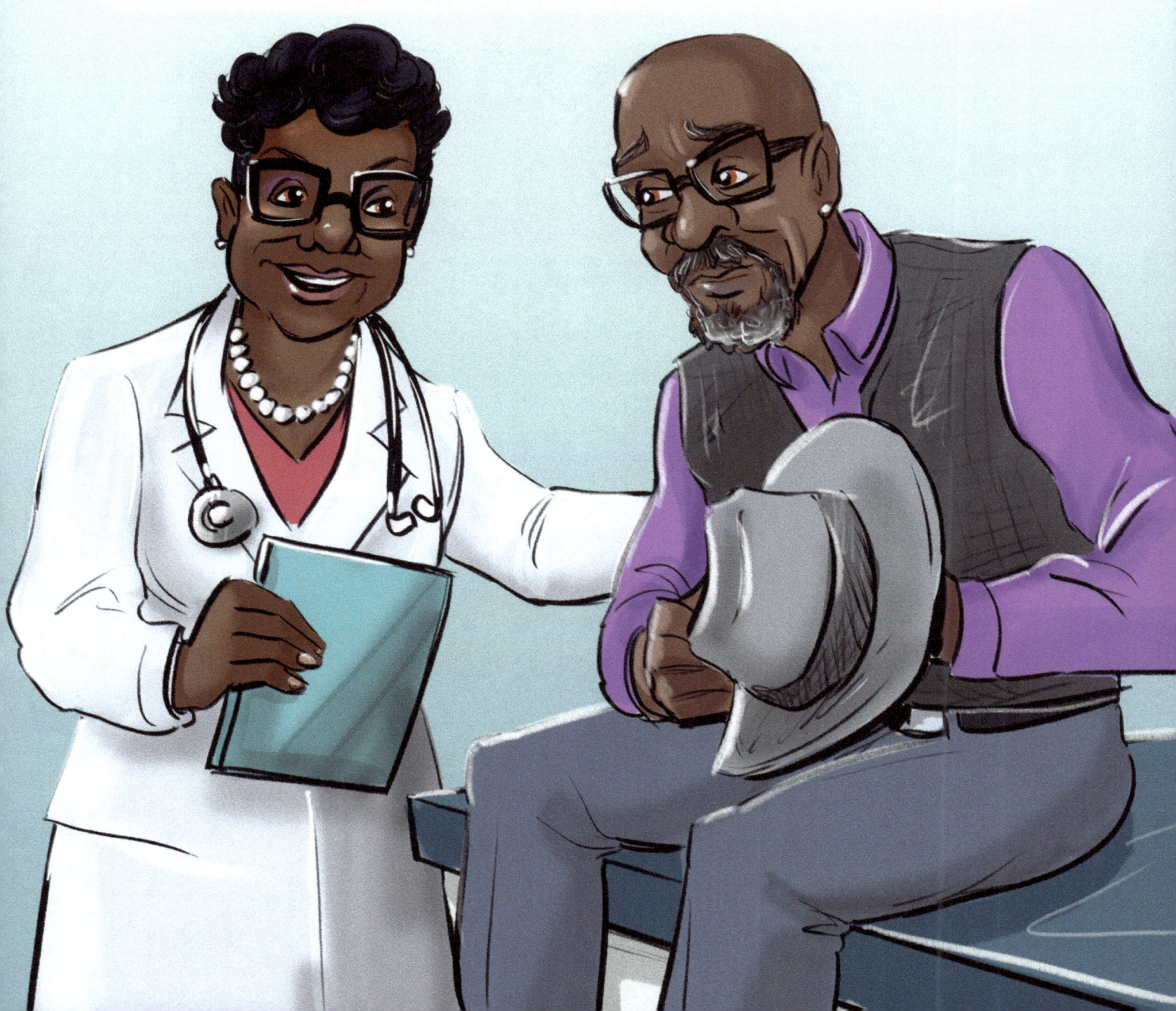

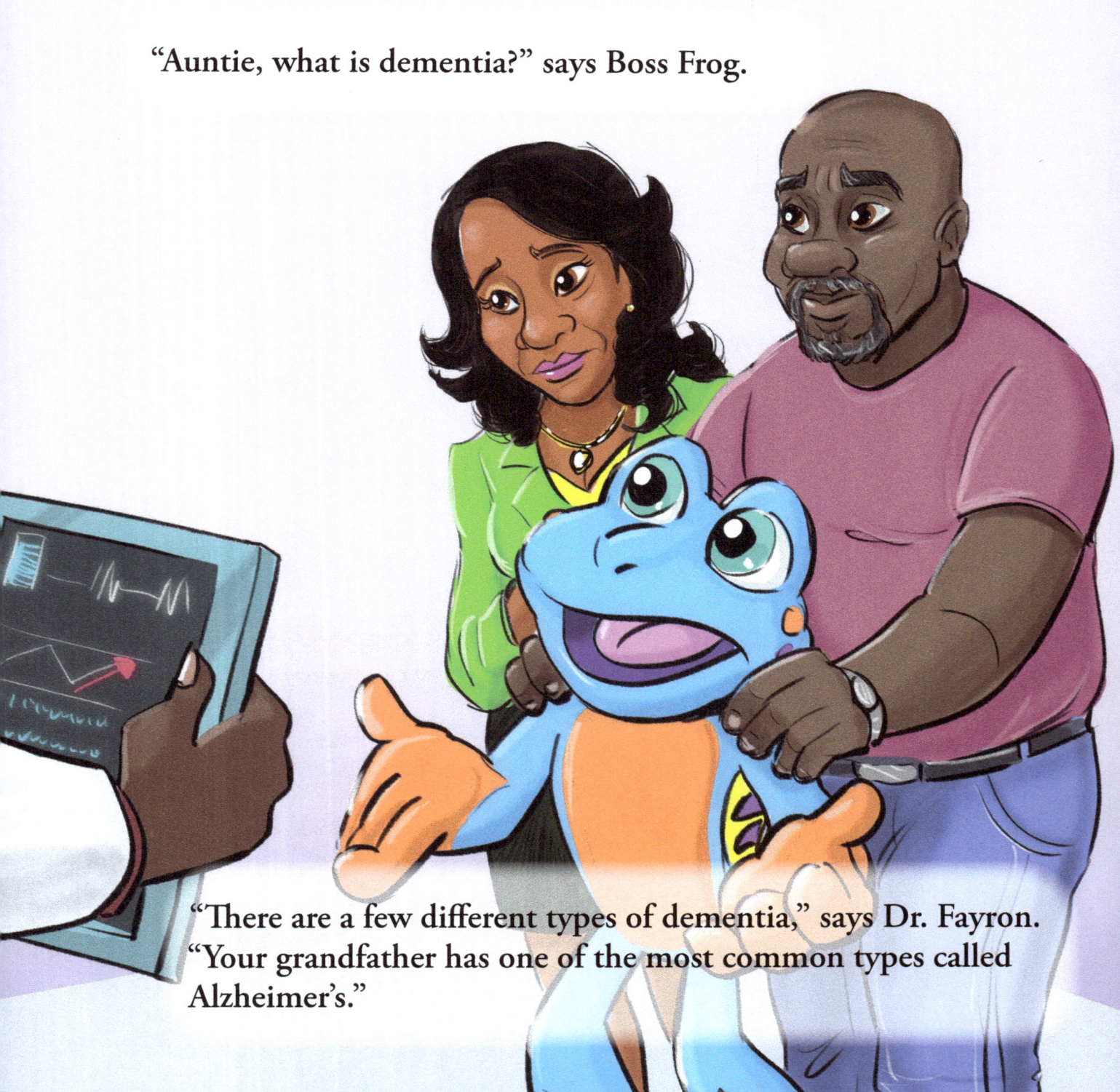

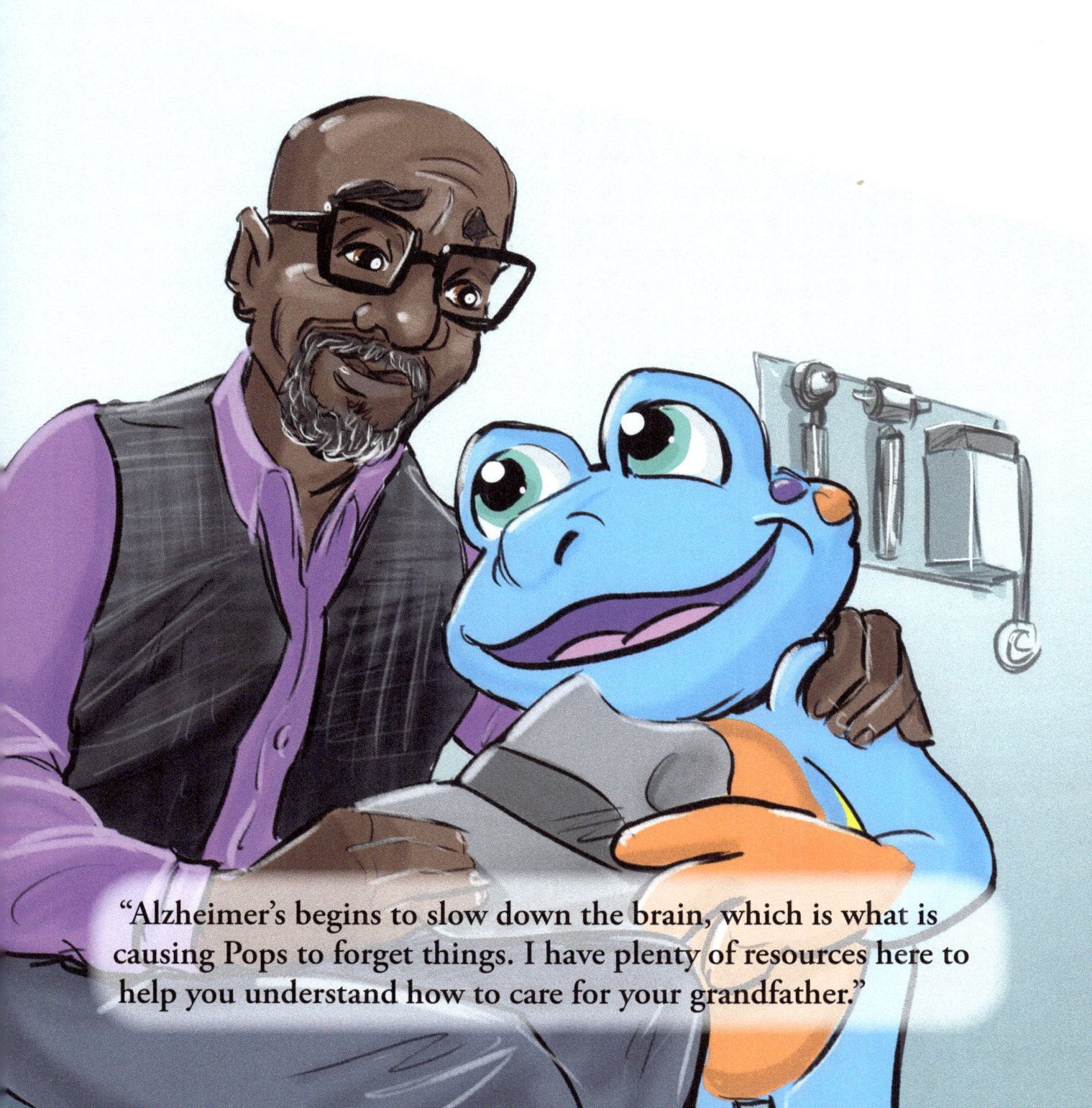

"Alzheimer's begins to slow down the brain, which is what is causing Pops to forget things. I have plenty of resources here to help you understand how to care for your grandfather."

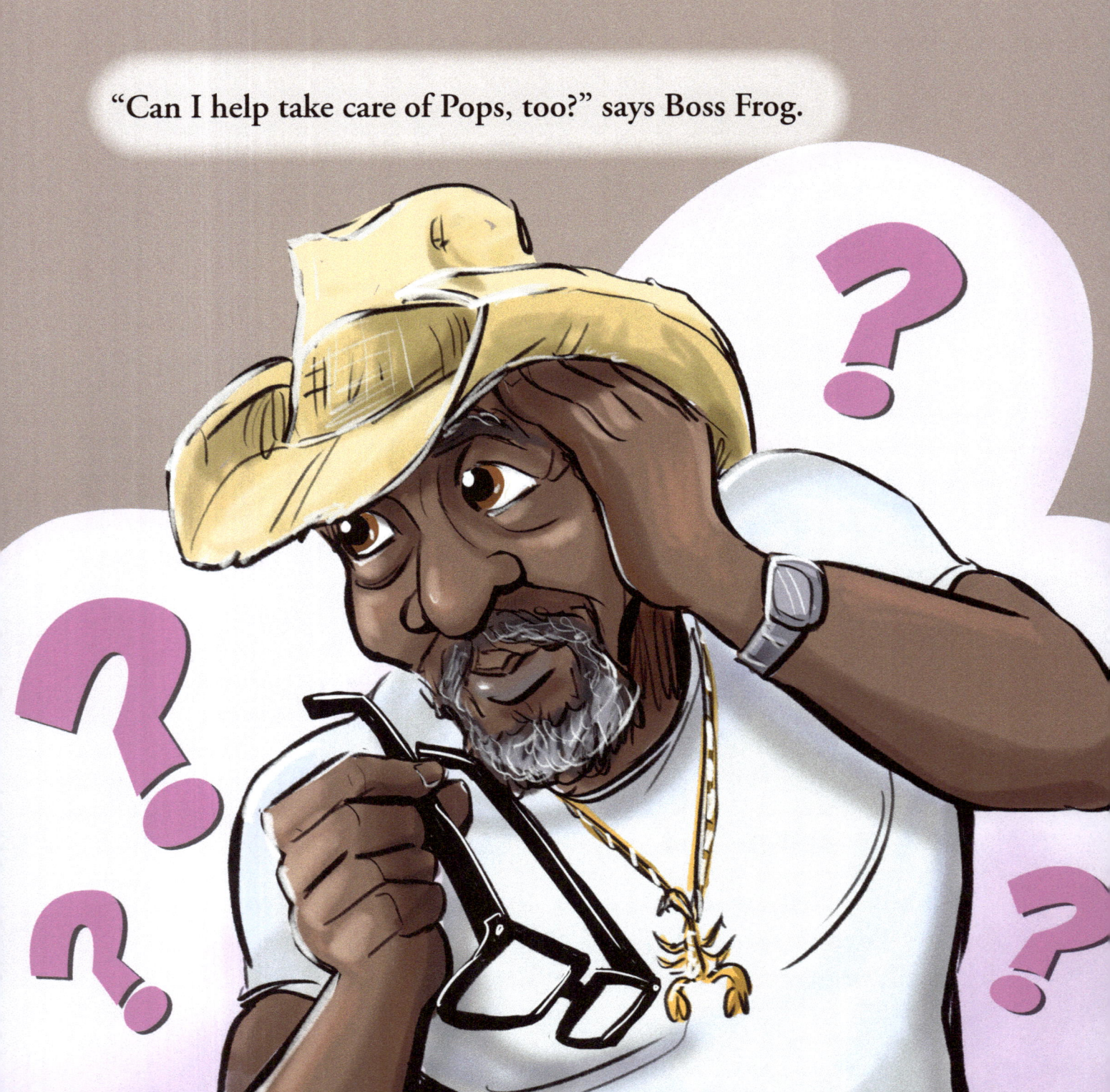

"Absolutely, Boss Frog! We love when our youth want to help. Youth caregivers play an important role in our families," says Dr. Fayron.

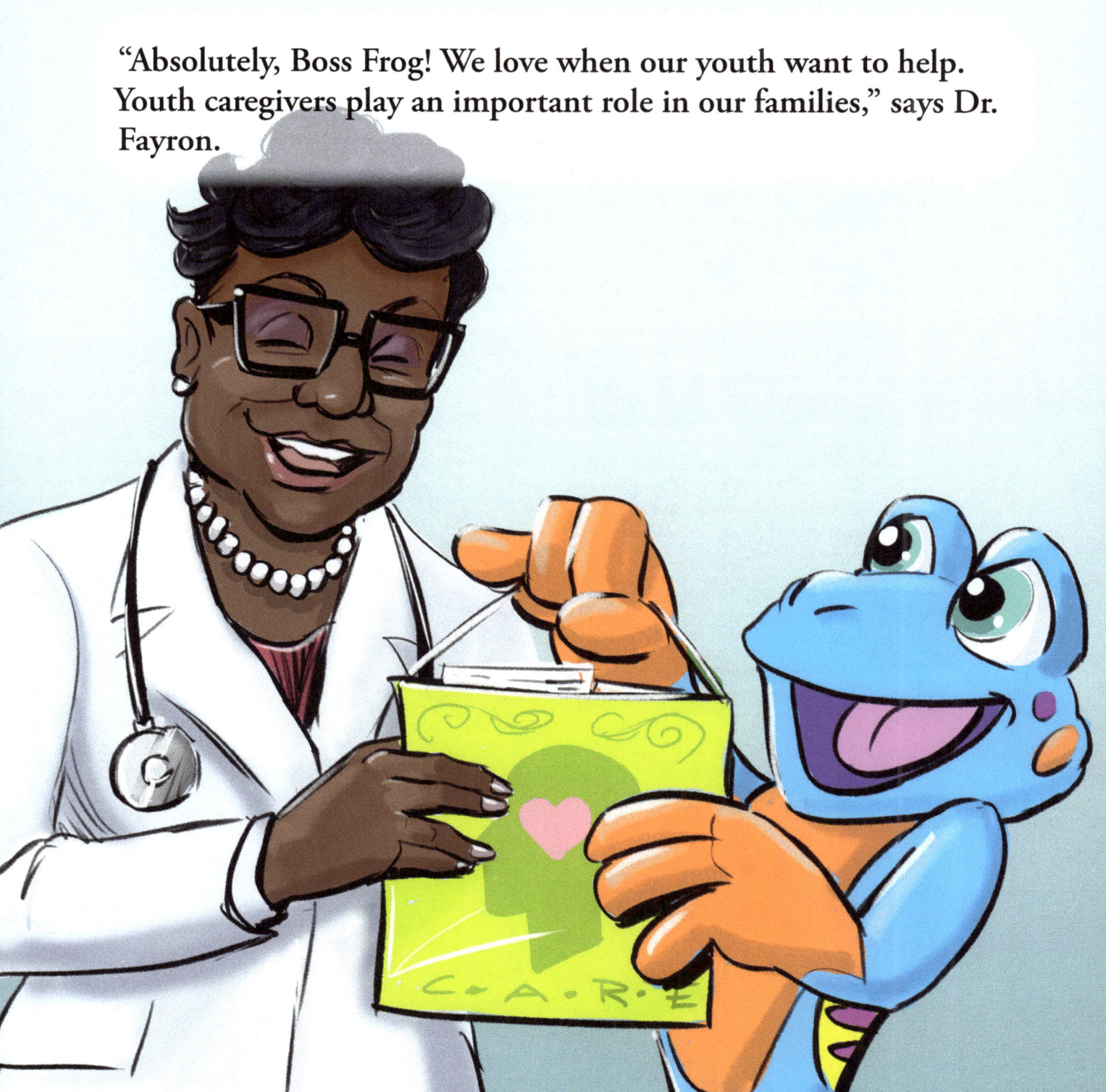

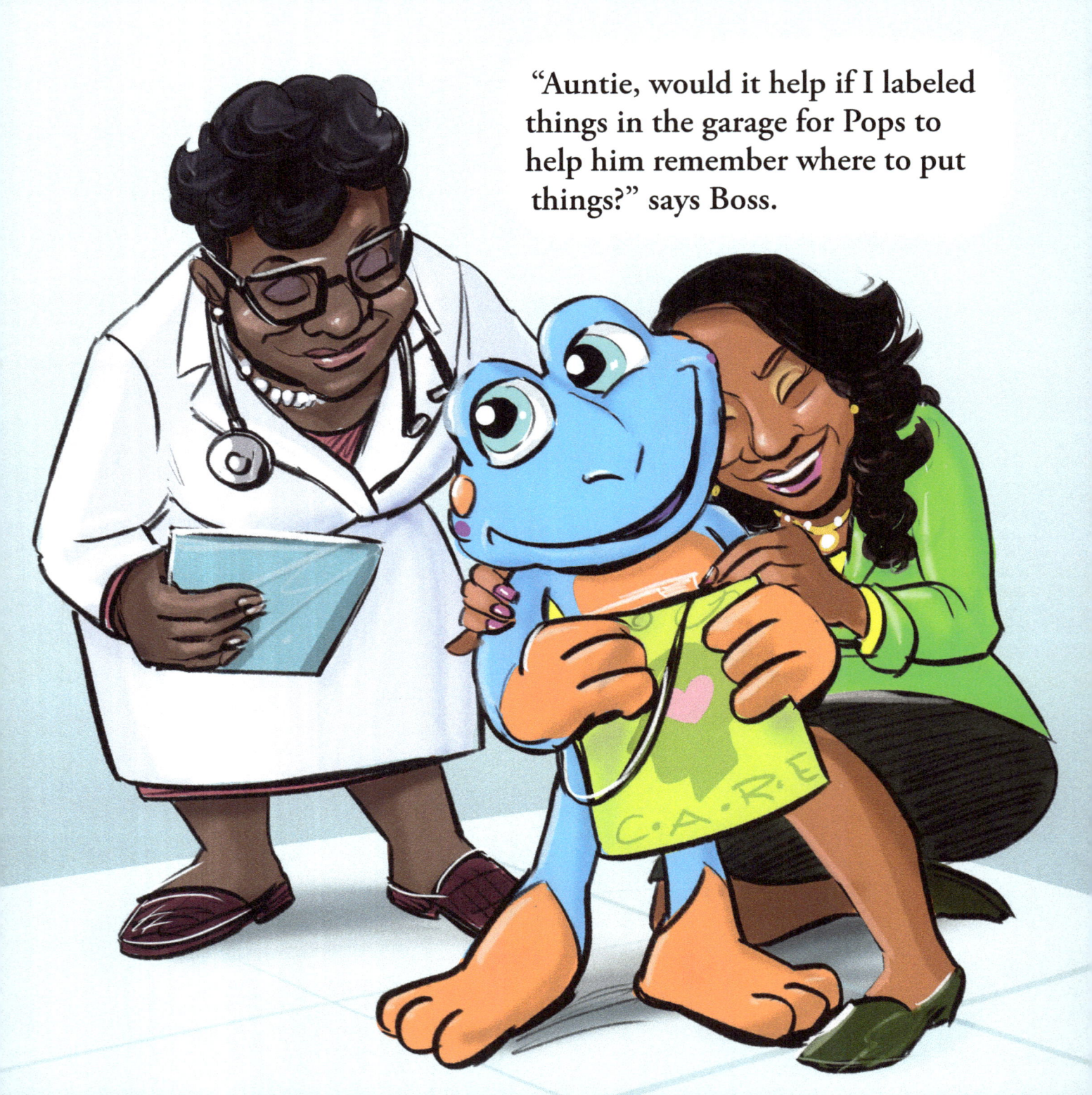

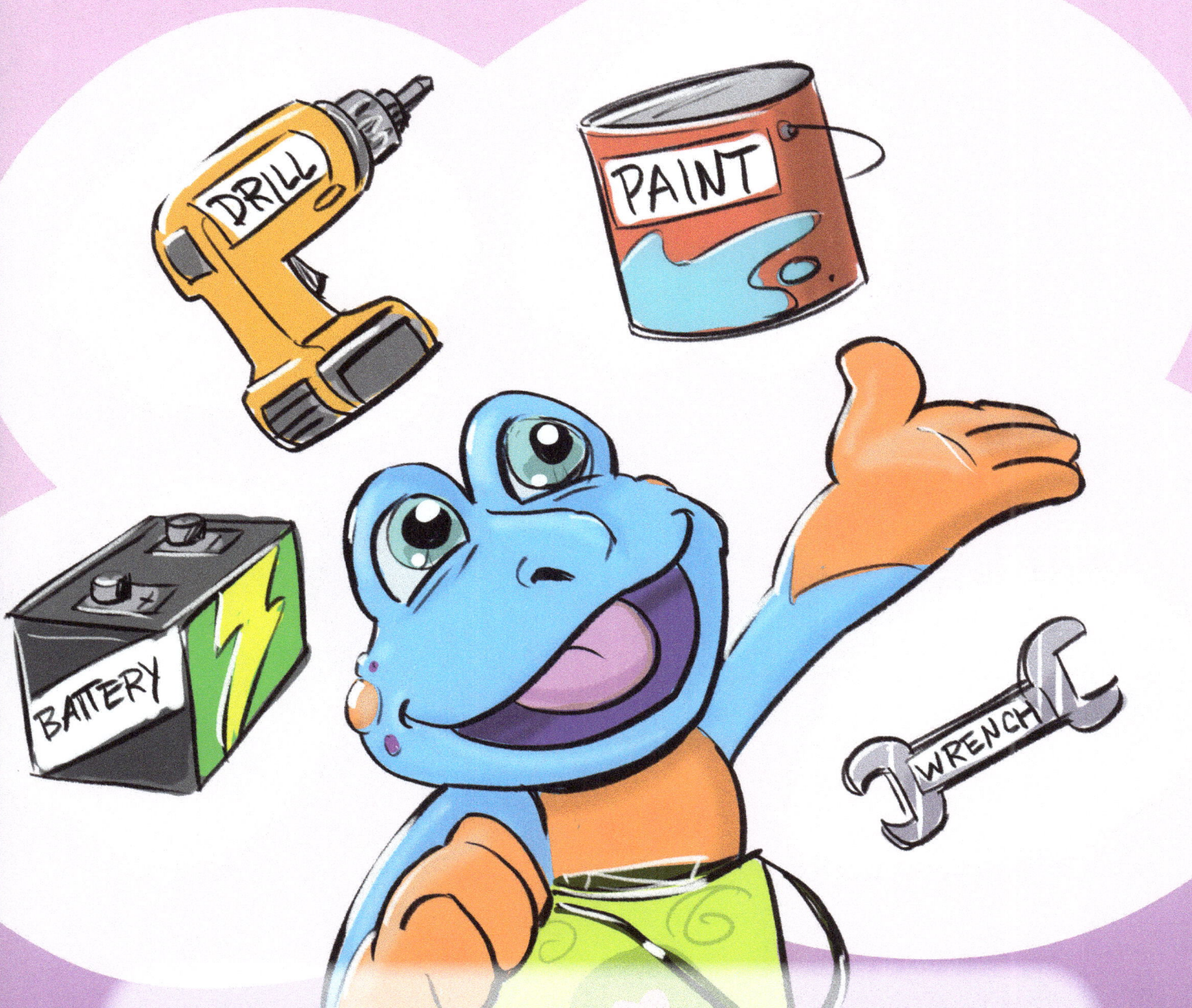

"Yes, nephew! That's a great idea! You can create a fun memory game for Pops and his tools once we get back home."

"Thank you, Dr. Fayron, for your help today. We appreciate all that you have done for our family," says Uncle Raul.

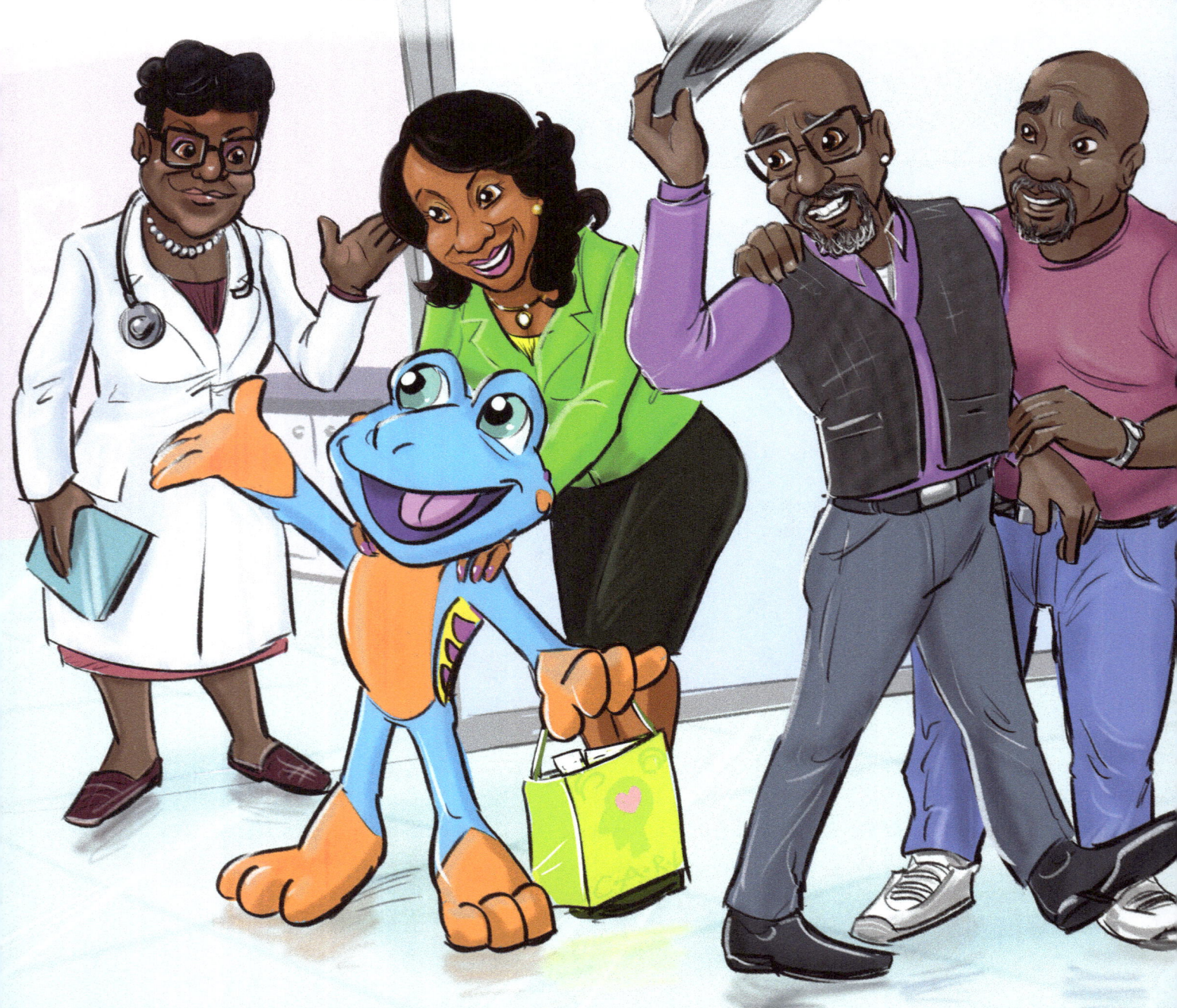

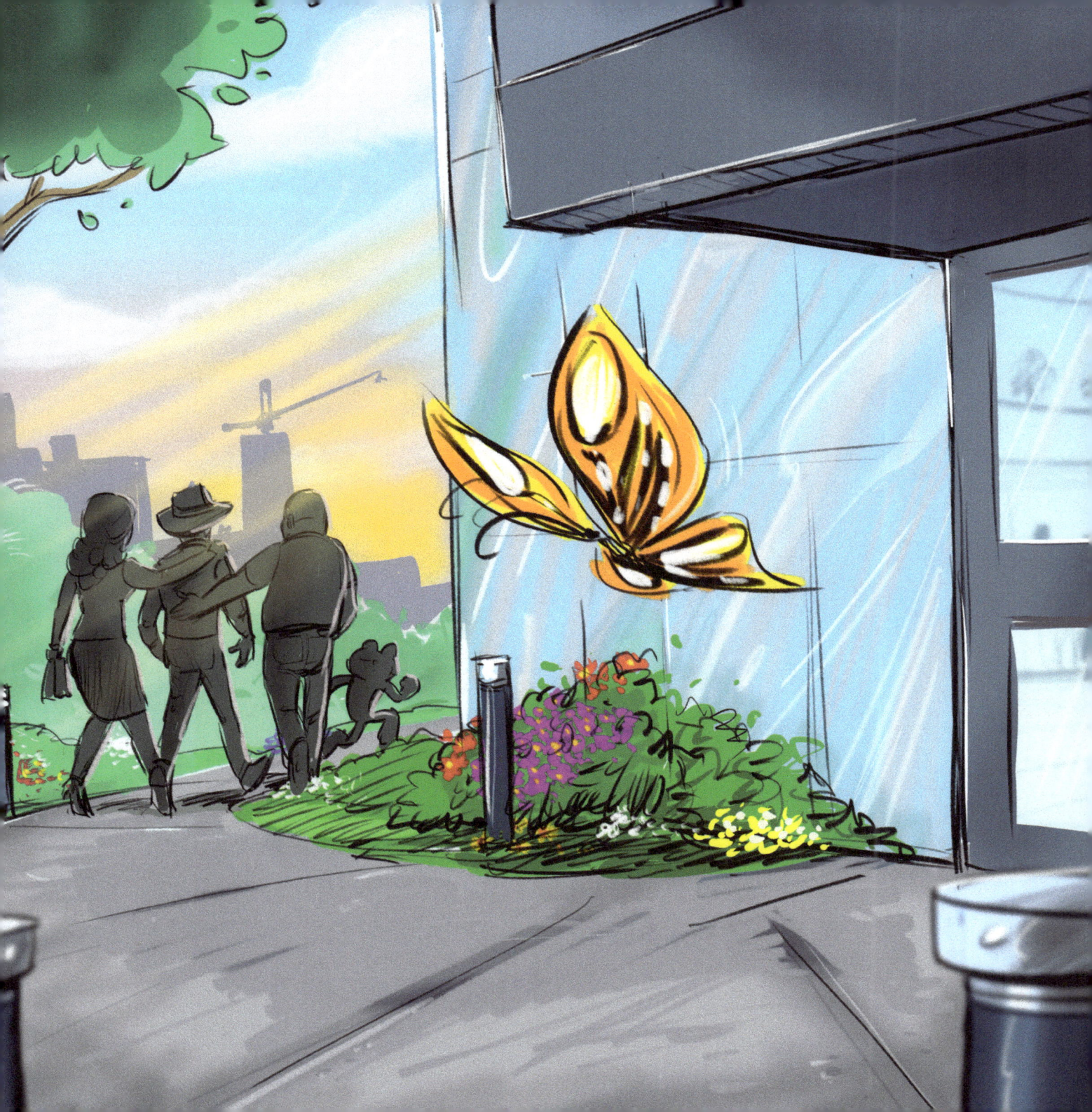

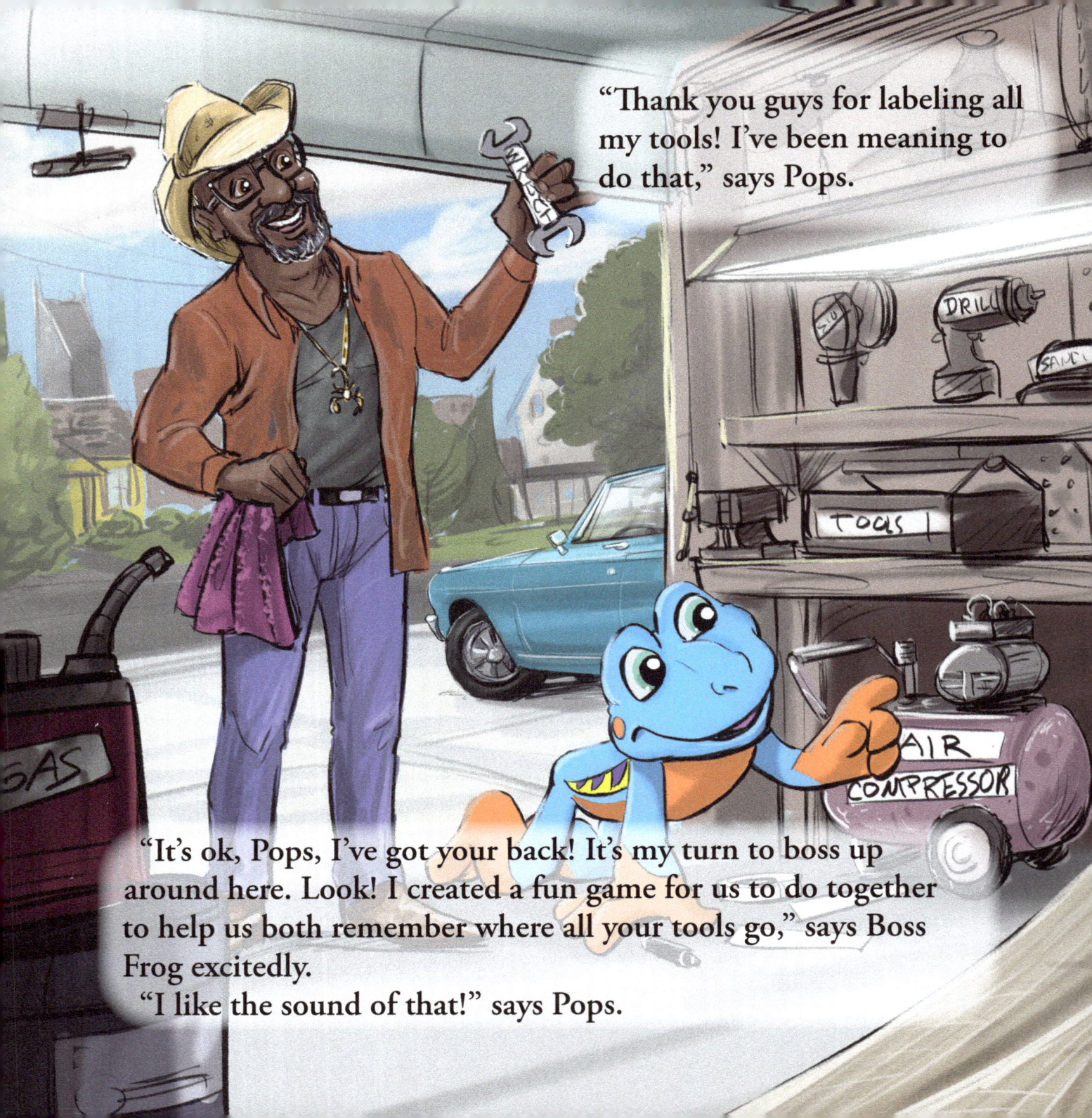

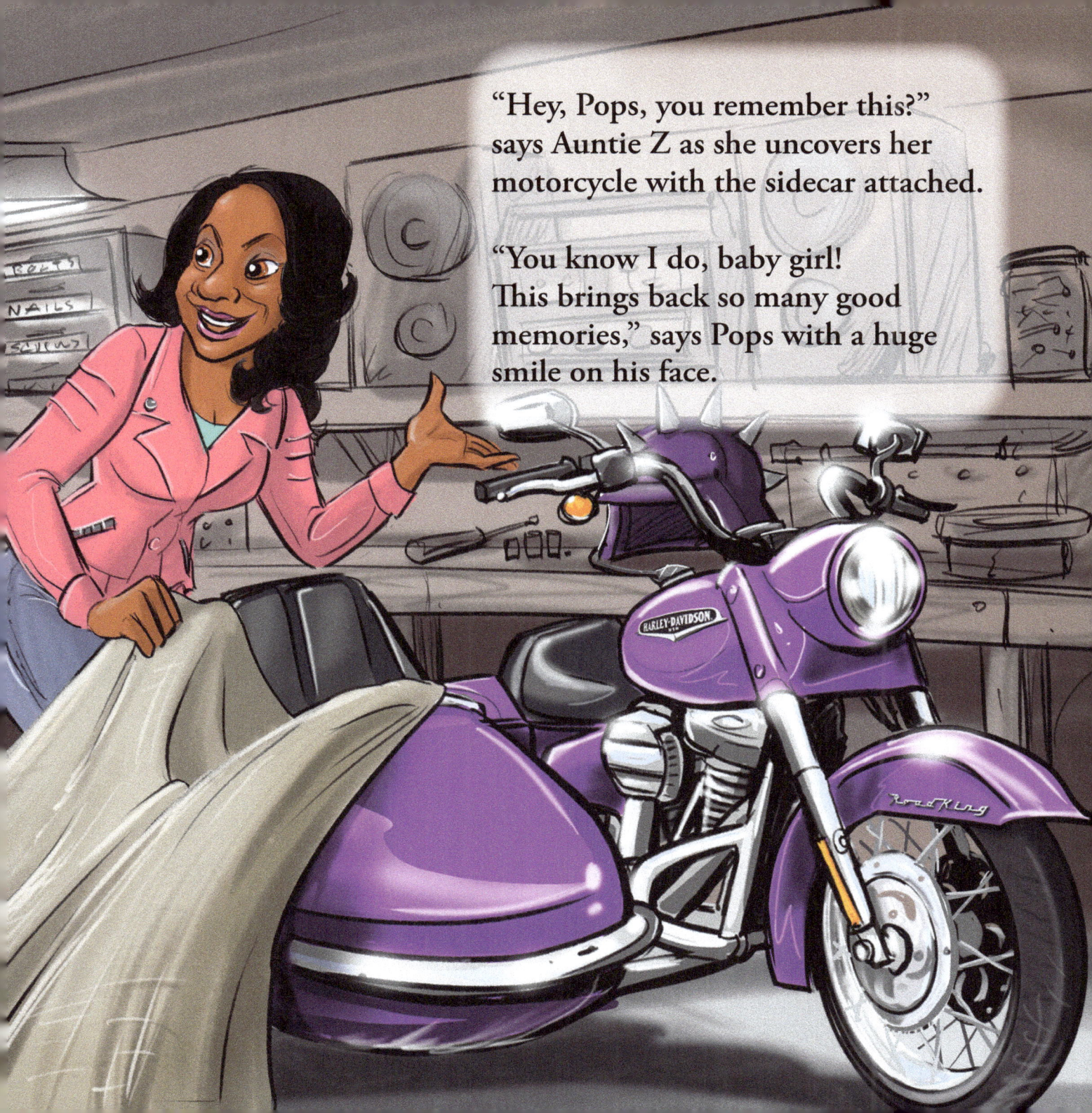

"All it needed was a little bit of this and a little bit of that!" they both said at the same time with a fist bump.

"I knew you wouldn't forget our motorcycles. Now, let's ride," says Auntie Z.

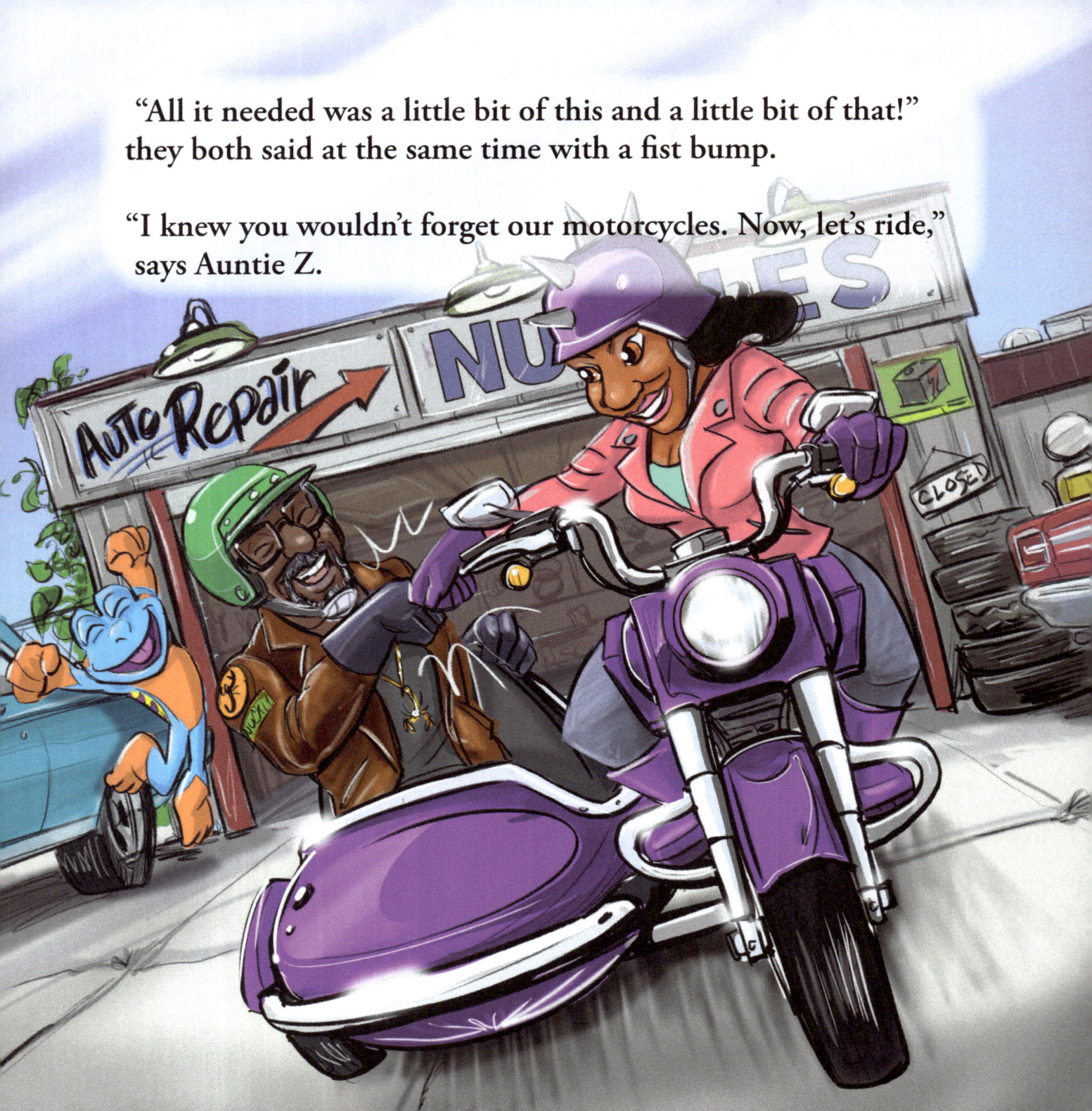

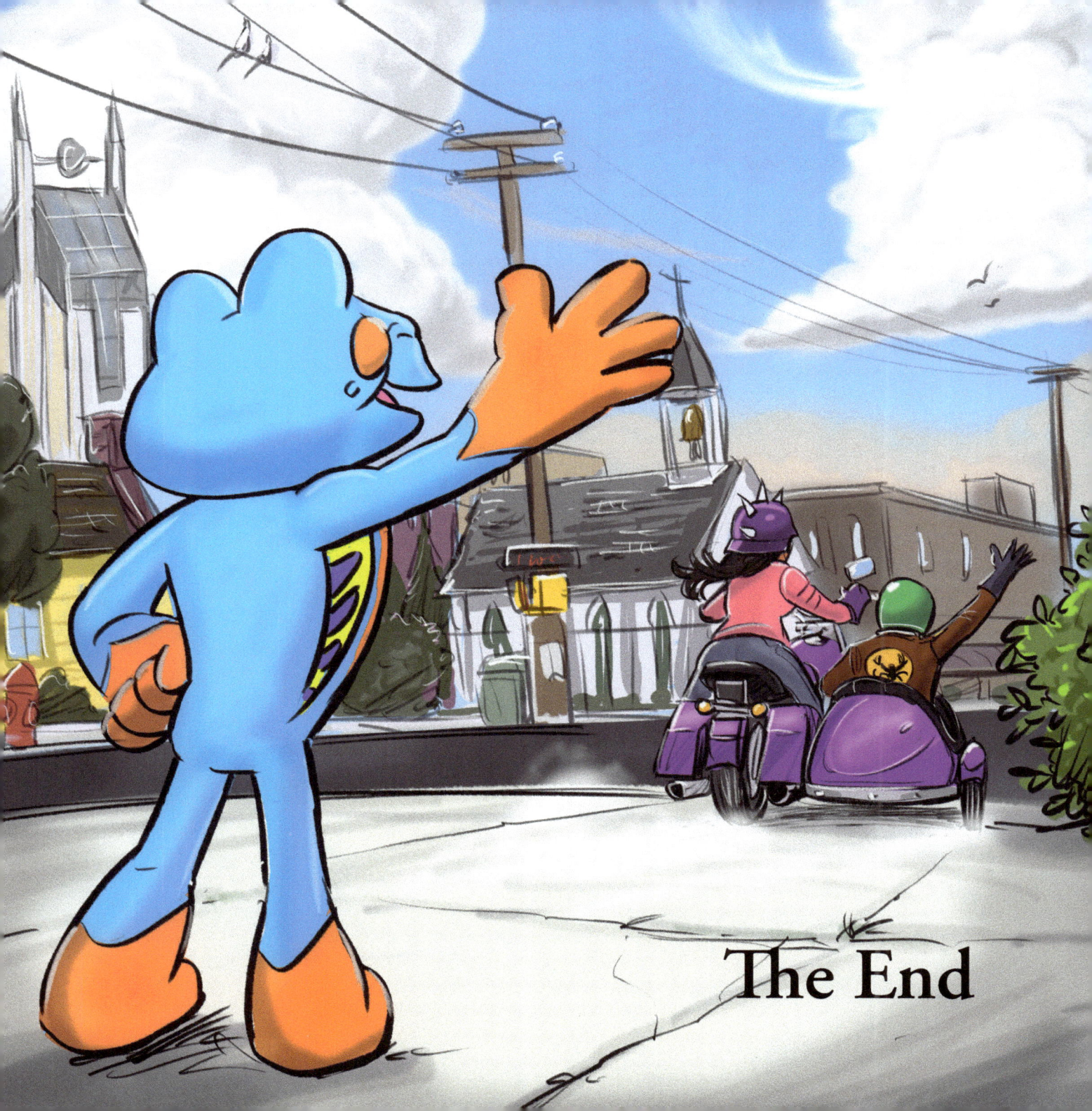

Resource Questions

1. What type of dementia does Pops have?

2. What does Pops keep in his garage?

3. What were some things Boss Frog noticed about Pops in the garage?

4. What did the family do before they started eating?

5. Just because we get older, does that mean we will get Alzheimer's?

6. What does Boss Frog do to help Pops remember where his tools go?

7. Who is Pops to Boss Frog?

Answers:

1. Alzheimer's

2. Cars, trucks, motorcycles, and tools

3. Boss Frog noticed that Pops was getting frustrated and confused.

4. The family said grace over food.

5. No, our age does not mean we will get Alzheimer's.

6. Boss Frog labeled all of Pops' tools.

7. Pops is Boss Frog's Grandpa.

Meet The Creator:
Xylina Cassandra

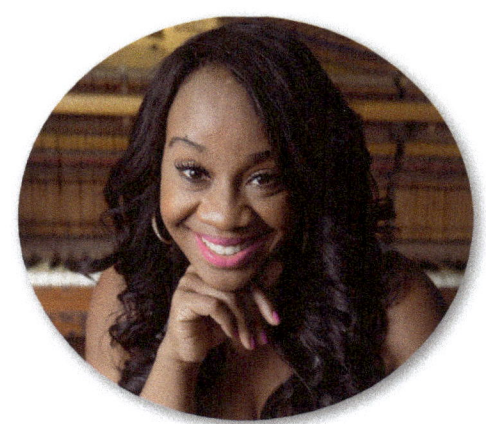

As an up-and-coming force in the industry, Xylina Cassandra is an author, certified Life Coach, CDP, CNA, a producer, singer, motorcyclist, and the creator of Boss Frog™.

As a CNA (Certified Nurse Assistant) and CDP, Certified by the National Council of Certified Dementia practitioners, Xylina combines her passion for the arts with health and wellness to create very unique intergenerational programs for seniors and their grandchildren.

Xylina has produced children's shows for over a decade. She created a self-confidence building drama enrichment program for grades K-8th called Artist 360. She is also featured on Oprah Winfrey's The Own Network on the award-winning series Green Leaf for two seasons. Xylina attended Stephens College in Columbia, Missouri, where she earned a Bachelor of Fine Arts degree in Theatre.

"So...why the name Ms. Z if your name starts with the letter 'X'?

Xylina (Pronounced ZU-LEENA): "Over the years, my students assumed my name started with the letter 'Z' and so the name Ms. Z stuck with me. And it doesn't bother me one bit." #MYLIFE was a promise I made to the God I serve to live my life in my purpose. It is my mission to keep that promise.

- Xylina Cassandra

Dr. Fayron Epps

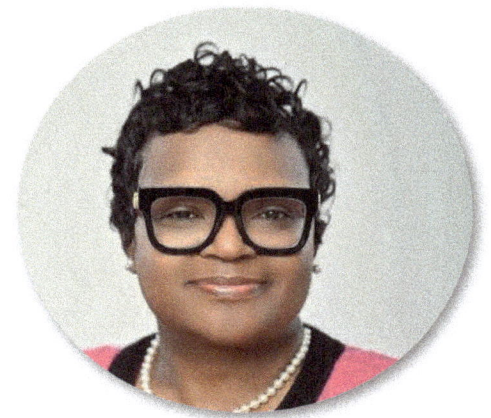

Dr. Fayron Epps is a distinguished nurse leader and researcher specializing in dementia care, family caregiving, and health disparities. She serves as Professor and holds the Karen and Ronald Herrmann Distinguished Chair in Caregiver Research at The University of Texas Health Science Center San Antonio School of Nursing.

Internationally recognized for her community-engaged scholarship, Dr. Fayron partners with faith communities to improve dementia care and expand access to culturally relevant resources. Her research centers on how faith-based organizations can serve as vital support systems for families and caregivers, particularly in underserved communities disproportionately affected by dementia. Dr. Fayron is the founder of Alter, the only nurse-led, dementia-friendly congregation program, and she oversees several psychoeducational and faith-based projects, such as "Beyond Box" and "Caregiving while Black."

Dr. Fayron is committed to bridging the gap between research and real-world impact, ensuring her work translates into meaningful change for the populations she serves. Her innovative contributions to health equity, dementia care, and community engagement have been recognized through numerous awards and national funding.

Dr. Fayron

Creating a Culture of Care

DrFayron.com
info@drfayron.com

Meet Boss Frog

Boss Frog is an Afro-Latino Tree Frog from Columbia who was raised in Gainesville, Georgia and mentored by his auntie, Ms. Z.

If you could describe Boss Frog, you'd say slightly self-indulgent, dramatic, urban, funny, and everyone knows he doesn't play about his nana! Boss Frog and his Auntie Z take on many adventures on their motorcycle, and together they sing, act, and dance.

Boss Frog educates on issues such as:

Mental health, Alzheimer's and Dementia, STEM, Health and Wellness, Literacy, Cancer, Child Obesity, Financial literacy, Bullying, Diversity and Inclusion, Dwarfism Awareness, Brain Health, Autism, and Motorcycle Safety.

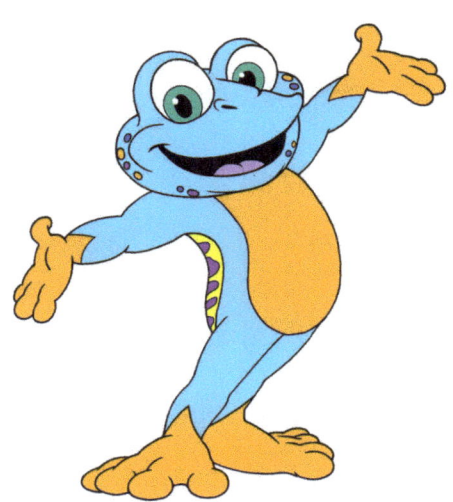

www.ingramcontent.com/pod-product-compliance
Lightning Source LLC
Chambersburg PA
CBHW040003040426
42337CB00032B/5205